Gestational Diabetes Cookbook for Newly Diagnosed

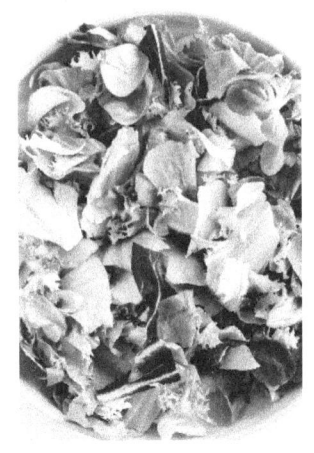

Lily Sablon, RDN

Legal Disclaimer

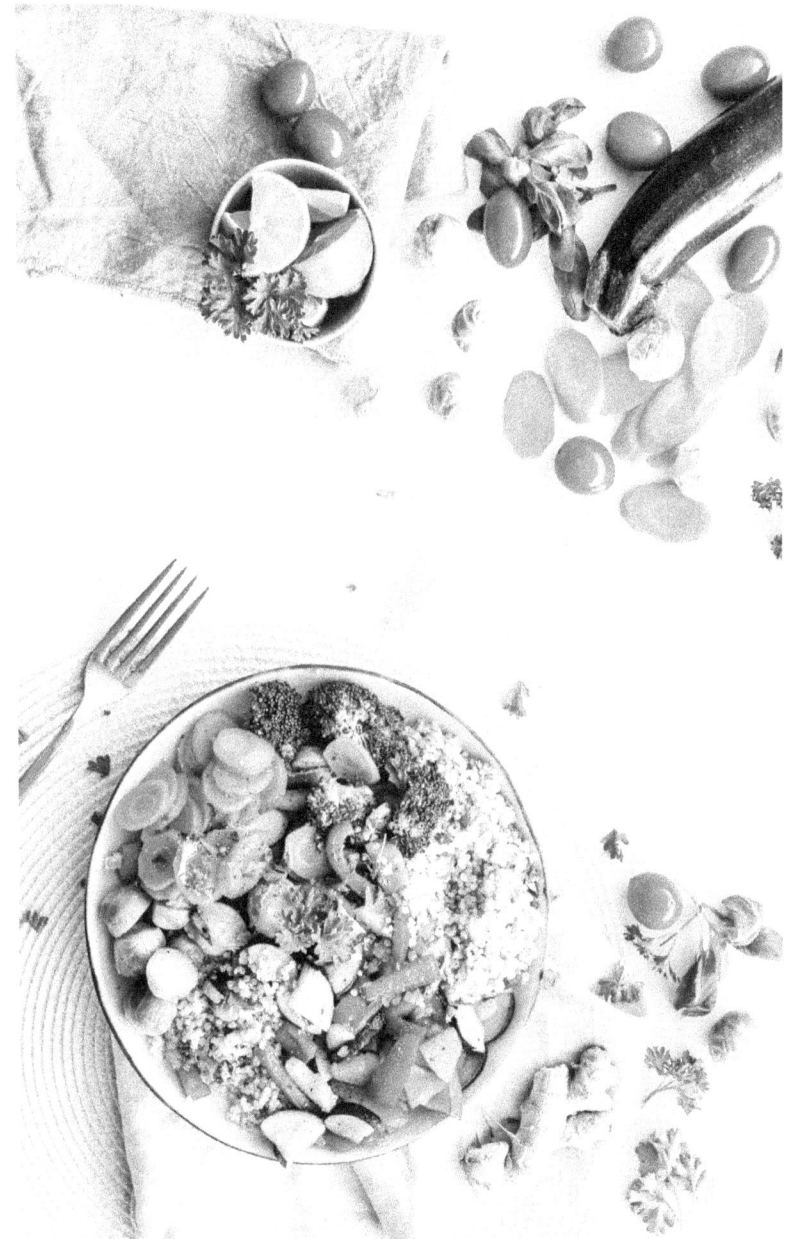

How is Gestational Diabetes Diagnosed?

Gestational diabetes is diagnosed with a blood test called a glucose challenge test. This test is usually done between 24 and 28 weeks of pregnancy. If you have an abnormal glucose challenge test, you will need to take a second test called a 3-hour glucose tolerance test.

How is Gestational Diabetes Managed?

Gestational diabetes can be managed with a healthy diet, exercise, and sometimes insulin. The goal of managing gestational diabetes is to keep your blood sugar levels in a healthy range. This will help to protect your baby from health problems such as birth defects, macrosomia (a baby that is too large for gestational age), and hypoglycemia (low blood sugar).

What are the Risks of Gestational Diabetes?

Gestational diabetes can increase the risk of the following health problems for both mother and baby:

- Preeclampsia
- Birth defects
- Macrosomia
- Hypoglycemia
- Cesarean section
- Type 2 diabetes later in life

Symptoms of Gestational Diabetes

There are often no symptoms of gestational diabetes. However, some women may experience the following symptoms:

- Increased thirst

- Increased hunger
- Frequent urination
- Fatigue
- Blurred vision
- Weight gain
- Vaginal yeast infection
- Headache

If you experience any of these symptoms, it is important to talk to your doctor. Gestational diabetes can be diagnosed with a simple blood test.

How Can I Prevent Gestational Diabetes?

There is no sure way to prevent gestational diabetes, but there are some things you can do to reduce your risk, such as:

- Maintaining a healthy weight before pregnancy
- Eating a healthy diet
- Exercising regularly
- Quitting smoking
- Getting regular prenatal care

If You Have Gestational Diabetes, What Can You Expect?

If you have gestational diabetes, you will need to see your doctor or midwife more often than women who do not have gestational diabetes. You will also need to have your blood sugar levels checked regularly. Your doctor or midwife will work with you to create a plan to manage your gestational diabetes. This plan may include diet, exercise, and insulin.

What Happens After My Baby Is Born?

After your baby is born, you will need to have your blood sugar levels checked regularly for several weeks. Your doctor or midwife will also monitor your baby for signs of hypoglycemia. Most women who have gestational diabetes do not have any long-term health problems. However, you are at an increased risk of developing type 2 diabetes later in life. It is important to talk to your doctor about how to reduce your risk of developing type 2 diabetes.

Gestational diabetes can be a challenging condition, but it is important to remember that you are not alone.

What to Eat with Gestational Diabetes

Tips & Benefits

Eating a healthy diet is an important part of managing gestational diabetes. By making smart food choices, you can help keep your blood sugar levels in a healthy range and reduce your risk of complications.

Here are some tips for what to eat with gestational diabetes:

- Choose whole grains over refined grains. Whole grains are a good source of fiber, which can help to slow down the absorption of sugar into your bloodstream.
- Choose lean protein sources. Lean protein sources, such as chicken, fish, beans, and tofu, can help you feel full and satisfied without raising your blood sugar levels.
- Choose low-fat dairy products. Low-fat dairy products, such as milk, yogurt, and cheese, are good sources of calcium and protein.

- Choose seasonal fruits and vegetables. Fruits and vegetables are a good source of vitamins, minerals, and fiber. Choose fresh, frozen, or canned fruits and vegetables without added sugar or syrup.
- Choose healthy fats. Healthy fats, such as olive oil, avocado, nuts, and seeds, can help to keep you feeling full and satisfied.
- Limit sugary drinks. Sugary drinks, such as soda, juice, and sports drinks, can raise your blood sugar levels quickly. Choose water, unsweetened tea, or coffee instead.
- Limit processed foods. Processed foods are often high in sugar, unhealthy fats, and sodium. Choose whole, unprocessed foods whenever possible.

Regular meals and snacks should be eaten throughout the day. This will assist in maintaining steady blood sugar levels. Try not to go extended periods without eating.

The Environmental Working Group, a nonprofit environmental watchdog group, examines data on pesticide residues provided by the U.S. Department of Agriculture and the Food and Drug Administration.

It generates a ranking of the top and worst pesticide doses discovered in industrial crops each year.

These lists might help you choose which foods are considered safe enough to be purchased conventionally and which should be purchased organically to reduce your exposure to pesticides. Although they are safe to purchase, these fruits and vegetables should still be carefully washed.

The list is updated annually, and you can find it online at EWG.org/FoodNews

If you are unsure about what to eat, talk to your doctor or a registered dietitian. They can help you create a personalized meal plan that meets your needs and helps you manage your gestational diabetes.

What to Avoid with Gestational Diabetes

Here are some foods and drinks that you should avoid if you have gestational diabetes:

Sugary drinks: Soda, juice, sports drinks, and sweetened tea and coffee

Processed foods: Packaged snacks, frozen meals, and fast food

White bread, pasta, and rice: These refined grains are digested quickly and can raise blood sugar levels

Simple carbohydrates: These foods are high in sugar and can also raise blood sugar levels quickly

Trans fats: These unhealthy fats are found in some processed foods and can raise cholesterol levels

Alcohol: Alcohol can raise blood sugar levels and can also have other negative effects on pregnancy

It is also important to limit your intake of saturated fat and cholesterol. These unhealthy fats can raise your risk of heart disease and other health problems.

Meal Planning for Gestational Diabetes

Meal planning for gestational diabetes can be tricky, but it doesn't have to be. By following these tips, you can create healthy and delicious meals that will help you manage your blood sugar levels and have a healthy pregnancy.

1. Choose whole grains over refined grains.

Whole grains are a good source of fiber, which can help to slow down the absorption of sugar into your bloodstream.

2. Choose lean protein sources.

Lean protein sources, such as chicken, fish, beans, and tofu, can help you feel full and satisfied without raising your blood sugar levels.

3. Choose low-fat dairy products.

Low-fat dairy products, such as milk, yogurt, and cheese, are a good source of calcium and protein.

4. Choose fruits and vegetables.

Fruits and vegetables are good sources of vitamins, minerals, and fiber. Choose fresh, frozen, or canned fruits and vegetables without added sugar or syrup.

5. Choose healthy fats.

Healthy fats, such as olive oil, avocado, nuts, and seeds, can help to keep you feeling full and satisfied.

6. Stop sugary drinks.

Sugary drinks, such as soda, juice, and sports drinks, can raise your blood sugar levels quickly. Choose water, unsweetened tea, or coffee instead.

7. Limit processed foods.

Processed foods are often high in sugar, unhealthy fats, and sodium. Choose whole, unprocessed foods whenever possible.

8. Read food labels carefully.

When you're shopping for food, be sure to read the labels carefully. Pay attention to the serving size, calories, and grams of carbohydrates.

9. Talk to your doctor or a registered dietitian.

If you're unsure about what to eat, talk to your doctor or a registered dietitian. They can help you create a personalized meal plan that meets your needs and helps you manage your gestational diabetes.

Here are some examples of healthy meals for gestational diabetes:

Breakfast:

- Oatmeal with berries and nuts
- Whole-wheat toast with peanut butter and banana
- Yogurt with fruit and granola
- Egg white omelet with vegetables

Lunch:

- Salad with grilled chicken or fish
- Soup and salad
- Sandwich on whole-wheat bread with lean protein, vegetables, and low-fat cheese
- Leftovers from dinner

Dinner:

- Grilled salmon with roasted vegetables
- Chicken stir-fry with brown rice
- Lentil soup
- Vegetarian chili

Snacks:

- Seasonal Fruit
- Yogurt

- Nuts
- Trail mix
- Hard-boiled eggs

By following these tips, you can create healthy and delicious meals that will help you manage your blood sugar levels and have a healthy pregnancy.

Kitchen Conversion Chart

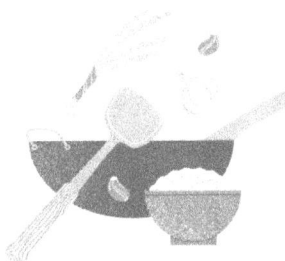

KITCHEN Conversion Guide

DRY MEASUREMENT

4 cups = 64 tbsp = 192 tsp		1/2 cup = 8 tbsp = 24 tsp
2 cups = 32 tbsp = 96 tsp		1/3 cup = 5 1/3 tbsp = 16 tsp
1 cup = 16 tbsp = 48 tsp		1/4 cup = 4 tbsp = 12 tsp
3/4 cup = 12 tbsp = 36 tsp		1/8 cup = 2 tbsp = 6 tsp
2/3 cup = 10 2/3 tbsp = 32 tsp		1/16 cup = 1 tbsp = 3 tsp

LIQUID MEASUREMENT

1 gallon = 4 quarts = 8 pints	1 cup = 1/2 pint = 16 tbsp
1/2 gallon = 2 quarts = 4 pints	1/2 cup = 8 tbsp = 24 tsp
1 quart = 1/4 gallon = 2 pints	1 oz = 1/4 cup = 4 tbsp
1 pint = 1/2 quart = 2 cups	

OVEN TEMPERATURE

500 F	=	260 C	=	10 Gas mark
475 F	=	240 C	=	9 Gas mark
450 F	=	230 C	=	8 Gas mark
425 F	=	220 C	=	7 Gas mark
400 F	=	200 C	=	6 Gas mark

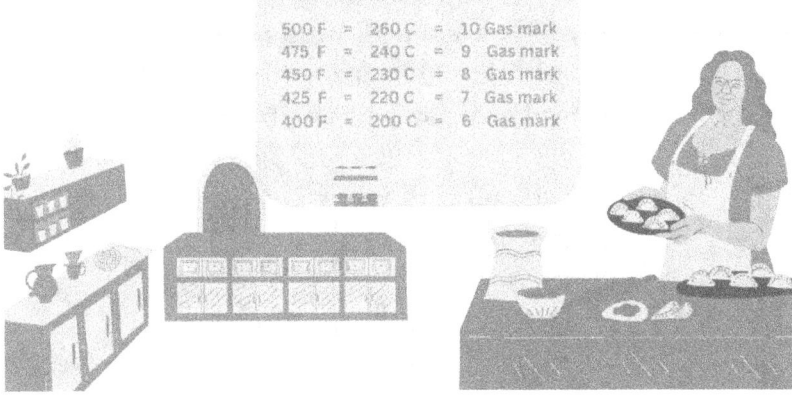

Snacks for Gestational Diabetes

Here are some healthy snacks for gestational diabetes:

- **Seasonal Fruit:** If it's not Berries and seasonal fruits, you shouldn't binge on fruits because you think it contains healthy Sugar. Sugar is Sugar no matter the Source, fruits contains fructose, very bad for you especially people with metabolic issues. Health professionals sing their praises in every ailment, oblivious to the fact that most of them are GMOs, filled with pesticides, force ripened, less fiber, less nutrients and loads of sugar. Fruits that are sugary should be avoided. Fruits that are less sugary should be taken liberally after it is washed with salt or vinegar. Many fruits are bioengineered, highly sweetened and ripened by chemicals, never binge on such.

- **Yogurt:** Yogurt is a good source of protein and calcium. It is also low in fat and calories. Choose plain yogurt and add your own fruit, nuts, or seeds.
- Nuts: Nuts are a good source of protein, fiber, and healthy fats. They are also low in carbohydrates. Some good choices include almonds, cashews, peanuts, pistachios, and walnuts.
- Trail mix: Trail mix is a great way to combine nuts, dried fruit, and whole-grain cereal. It is a portable and satisfying snack.
- Hard-boiled eggs: Hard-boiled eggs are a good source of protein and choline. They are also low in calories and carbohydrates.

It is important to choose snacks that are low in sugar and carbohydrates. These snacks will help to keep your blood sugar levels stable.

Recipes for Gestational Diabetes

Breakfast Recipes

Oatmeal with berries and nuts

Ingredients:

- 1 cup rolled oats
- 1 cup water
- 1 cup milk (any type)
- 1/2 teaspoon ground cinnamon
- 1/4 teaspoon salt
- 1/4 cup fresh or frozen berries

- 1/4 cup chopped nuts (walnuts, almonds, or pecans)

Instructions:

1. In a medium saucepan, combine oats, water, milk, cinnamon, and salt. Bring to a boil over medium heat, then reduce heat to low and simmer for 5 minutes, or until oats are cooked through.
2. Stir in berries and nuts. Serve immediately.

Total time: 10 minutes

Servings: 4

Tips:

- For a creamier oatmeal, use half milk and half water.
- Add a dollop of yogurt or peanut butter for extra protein.
- Top with your favorite fruit or nuts.

This recipe is a great way to start your day with a healthy and satisfying breakfast. Oats are a good source of fiber, which can help to keep your blood sugar levels stable. The berries are a good source of vitamins and minerals, and the nuts are a good source of protein and healthy fats.

Whole-wheat toast with peanut butter and banana

Ingredients:

- 2 slices whole-wheat bread
- 2 tablespoons peanut butter
- 1 banana, sliced

Instructions:

1. Toast the bread.

2. Spread peanut butter on one slice of toast.
3. Top with sliced banana.
4. Serve immediately.

Total time: 5 minutes

Servings: 2

Tips:

- Use natural peanut butter, which has no added sugar.
- Choose a banana that is ripe but not overripe.
- Add a drizzle of honey or maple syrup for sweetness.

This recipe is a quick and easy breakfast option that is perfect for people with gestational diabetes. Whole-wheat bread is a good source of fiber, which can help keep blood sugar levels stable. The peanut butter is a good source of protein and healthy fats, and the banana is a good source of potassium and vitamin C.

Yogurt with fruit and granola

Ingredients:

- 1 cup of plain yogurt
- 1/2 cup fresh or frozen fruit (such as berries, peaches, or mango)
- 1/4 cup granola

Instructions:

1. In a bowl, combine yogurt, fruit, and granola.
2. Stir until combined.
3. Serve immediately.

Total time: 5 minutes

Servings: 2

Tips:

- Use plain yogurt, which is lower in sugar than flavored yogurt.

- Choose fresh or frozen fruit that is low in sugar.
- Use a granola that is low in sugar and fat.

This recipe is a quick and easy breakfast option that is perfect for people with gestational diabetes. Yogurt is a good source of protein and calcium, and fruit is a good source of vitamins and minerals. The granola adds a bit of crunch and flavor.

Egg white omelet with vegetables

Ingredients:

- 6 egg whites
- 1/2 cup chopped vegetables (such as onions, peppers, mushrooms, or spinach)

- 1/4 teaspoon salt
- 1/8 teaspoon black pepper
- 1 tablespoon olive oil

Instructions:

1. In a bowl, whisk together the egg whites, vegetables, salt, and pepper.
2. Heat the olive oil in a nonstick skillet over medium heat.
3. Pour the egg mixture into the skillet and cook, stirring occasionally, until the eggs are set.
4. Serve immediately.

Total time: 10 minutes

Servings: 2

Tips:

- Use low-fat or fat-free egg whites.
- Choose vegetables that are low in carbohydrates.
- Season the omelet to taste with your favorite herbs and spices.

This recipe is a healthy and delicious breakfast option that is perfect for people with gestational diabetes. The egg whites are a good source of protein, and the vegetables are a good source of vitamins and minerals. The omelet is also low in carbohydrates and calories.

Scrambled eggs with spinach and avocado

Ingredients:

- 2 large eggs
- 1/4 cup milk
- 1/4 teaspoon salt
- 1/8 teaspoon black pepper
- 1/2 cup chopped spinach
- 1/4 avocado, diced

Instructions:

1. In a bowl, whisk together the eggs, milk, salt, and pepper.
2. Heat a nonstick skillet over medium heat.
3. Add the spinach to the skillet and cook until wilted, about 2 minutes.
4. Pour the egg mixture into the skillet and cook, stirring occasionally, until the eggs are set.
5. Stir in the avocado and serve immediately.

Total time: 10 minutes

Servings: 2

Tips:

- Use low-fat or fat-free milk.
- Choose spinach that is low in carbohydrates.
- Season the eggs to taste with your favorite herbs and spices.

This recipe is a healthy and delicious breakfast option that is perfect for people with gestational diabetes. The eggs are a good source of protein, and the spinach and avocado are a good source of vitamins and minerals. The eggs are also low in carbohydrates and calories.

Tofu scramble

Ingredients:

- 1 block extra-firm tofu, crumbled
- 1 tablespoon olive oil
- 1/2 onion, chopped
- 1 red bell pepper, chopped
- 1/2 teaspoon turmeric
- 1/4 teaspoon garlic powder
- 1/4 teaspoon salt
- 1/8 teaspoon black pepper
- 1/4 cup chopped fresh parsley

Instructions:

1. Heat the olive oil in a large skillet over medium heat.
2. Add the onion and bell pepper and cook until softened, about 5 minutes.
3. Add the tofu, turmeric, garlic powder, salt, and pepper and cook, stirring occasionally, until the tofu is heated through, about 5 minutes.
4. Stir in the parsley and serve immediately.

Total time: 15 minutes

Servings: 4

Tips:

- For a creamier scramble, add a splash of soy milk or water.
- Add your favorite vegetables, such as mushrooms, spinach, or zucchini.
- Season the scramble to taste with your favorite herbs and spices.

This recipe is a healthy and delicious breakfast option that is perfect for people with gestational diabetes. The tofu is a good source of protein, and the vegetables are a good source of vitamins and minerals. The scramble is also low in carbohydrates and calories.

Whole-wheat pancakes with fruit and syrup

Ingredients:

- 1 cup whole-wheat flour
- 1 teaspoon baking powder
- 1/2 teaspoon baking soda
- 1/4 teaspoon salt
- 1 egg
- 1 cup milk

- 1 tablespoon oil
- 1/2 cup berries, such as blueberries, raspberries, or strawberries
- 1/4 cup maple syrup

Instructions:

1. In a large bowl, whisk together the flour, baking powder, baking soda, and salt.
2. In a separate bowl, whisk together the egg, milk, and oil.
3. Add the wet ingredients to the dry ingredients and whisk until just combined.
4. Fold in the berries.
5. Heat a lightly oiled griddle or frying pan over medium heat.
6. Pour 1/4 cup of batter onto the hot griddle for each pancake.
7. Cook for 2-3 minutes per side, or until golden brown.
8. Serve immediately with maple syrup.

Total time: 20 minutes

Servings: 4

Tips:

- Use fresh or frozen berries.
- If you don't have whole-wheat flour, you can use all-purpose flour. Just add 1/4 teaspoon more baking powder.
- To make your own maple syrup, boil 1 cup of maple sugar or maple syrup over medium heat for 10-15 minutes, or until it thickens.

This recipe is a healthy and delicious breakfast option that is perfect for people with gestational diabetes. The pancakes are made with whole-wheat flour, which is a good source of fiber, and the fruit is a good source of vitamins and minerals. The pancakes are also low in carbohydrates and calories.

Waffles with fruit and whipped cream

Ingredients:

- 1 cup whole wheat flour
- 1 teaspoon baking powder
- 1/2 teaspoon baking soda
- 1/4 teaspoon salt
- 1 egg
- 1 cup unsweetened almond milk
- 1 tablespoon vegetable oil
- 1 teaspoon vanilla extract
- 1/2 cup fresh fruit, such as berries, sliced bananas, or peaches
- 1/4 cup whipped cream

Instructions:

1. Preheat your waffle iron according to the manufacturer's instructions.
2. In a large bowl, whisk together the flour, baking powder, baking soda, and salt.
3. In a separate bowl, whisk together the egg, almond milk, oil, and vanilla extract.

4. Add the wet ingredients to the dry ingredients and whisk until just combined.
5. Pour 1/4 cup of batter onto the hot waffle iron for each waffle.
6. Cook according to the manufacturer's instructions, or until golden brown.
7. Repeat steps 5 and 6 until all of the batter is used.
8. Serve the waffles immediately with fresh fruit and whipped cream.

Total time: 20 minutes

Servings: 4

Tips:

- For a sweeter waffle, add an extra tablespoon of sugar to the batter.
- If you don't have a waffle iron, you can make these waffles in a large skillet over medium heat. Just cook for 2-3 minutes per side, or until golden brown.

- Use your favorite fresh fruit in this recipe. Some other good options include strawberries, raspberries, blueberries, peaches, or mangoes.
- If you don't have whipped cream, you can use yogurt or ice cream instead.

Smoothie bowl with berries, yogurt, and nuts

Ingredients:

- 1 cup frozen berries (such as blueberries, raspberries, or strawberries)
- 1 cup plain Greek yogurt
- 1/2 cup milk of choice
- 1 tablespoon nut butter

- 1 teaspoon honey or maple syrup (optional)
- 1/4 cup chopped nuts (such as almonds, walnuts, or pecans)

Instructions:

1. Add all of the ingredients to a blender and blend until smooth.
2. Pour the smoothie into a bowl and top with your favorite toppings, such as granola, fruit, or nuts.
3. Enjoy!

Total time: 5 minutes

Servings: 1

Tips:

- Use frozen berries to make your smoothie extra cold.

- If you don't have milk of choice, you can use water or another type of milk.
- If you don't have honey or maple syrup, you can leave it out or use a sugar-free alternative.
- Choose your favorite nuts and toppings to make your smoothie bowl your own.

Omelet muffins

Ingredients:

- 12 muffin tins
- 1 tablespoon cooking spray
- 1/2 cup chopped onion
- 1/2 cup chopped green bell pepper
- 1/2 cup chopped mushrooms
- 1/2 cup shredded cheddar cheese
- 6 large eggs
- 1/4 cup milk

- 1/4 teaspoon salt
- 1/4 teaspoon black pepper

Instructions:

1. Preheat the oven to 350 degrees F (175 degrees C).
2. Grease the muffin tins with cooking spray.
3. In a large bowl, combine the onion, green bell pepper, mushrooms, and cheese.
4. In a separate bowl, whisk together the eggs, milk, salt, and pepper.
5. Pour the egg mixture into the muffin tins.
6. Top with the vegetable mixture.
7. Bake for 20-25 minutes, or until the eggs are set.
8. Let cool for a few minutes before serving.

Total time: 30 minutes

Servings: 12

Tips:

- You can use any type of vegetables in this recipe, such as broccoli, spinach, or zucchini.
- If you don't have cheddar cheese, you can use any type of shredded cheese.
- If you want a spicier omelet, you can add a pinch of cayenne pepper to the egg mixture.

Breakfast burritos

Ingredients:

- 2 large whole-wheat tortillas
- 1/2 cup cooked black beans
- 1/4 cup shredded cheddar cheese
- 1/4 cup chopped cooked vegetables, such as onions, peppers, or mushrooms
- 1/4 cup salsa
- 1/4 teaspoon salt
- 1/4 teaspoon black pepper

Instructions:

1. Preheat the oven to 350 degrees F (175 degrees C).
2. In a bowl, combine the black beans, cheese, vegetables, salsa, salt, and pepper.
3. Divide the mixture evenly between the two tortillas.
4. Roll up the tortillas and place them seam-side down on a baking sheet.

5. Bake for 10-12 minutes, or until the tortillas are heated through and the cheese is melted.
6. Cut the burritos in half and enjoy!

Total time: 20 minutes

Servings: 2

Tips:

- You can use any type of cooked beans in this recipe, such as pinto beans or kidney beans.
- You can also use any type of vegetables in this recipe, such as broccoli, spinach, or zucchini.
- If you don't have salsa, you can use ketchup or hot sauce.
- If you want a spicier burrito, you can add a pinch of cayenne pepper to the filling.

Ingredients:

- 2 whole-wheat English muffins
- 2 slices turkey bacon
- 2 eggs
- 1/4 cup shredded cheddar cheese
- 1/4 teaspoon salt
- 1/4 teaspoon black pepper

Instructions:

1. Cook the turkey bacon in a skillet over medium heat until crisp.
2. While the bacon is cooking, whisk the eggs together in a bowl.
3. Season the eggs with salt and pepper.
4. Once the bacon is cooked, remove it from the skillet and set it aside.
5. Add the eggs to the skillet and cook until they are set.
6. To assemble the sandwiches, spread a layer of cheese on each English muffin half.

7. Top with the cooked eggs, turkey bacon, and a sprinkle of salt and pepper.
8. Close the sandwiches and enjoy!

Tips:

- If you don't have turkey bacon, you can use regular bacon, but be sure to drain off any excess fat before adding the eggs.
  - You can also use other types of cheese, such as Swiss or Monterey Jack.
  - If you want a spicier sandwich, you can add a pinch of cayenne pepper to the eggs.

Total time: 10 minutes

Servings: 2

Yogurt parfaits

Ingredients:

- 1 cup plain yogurt
- 1/2 cup fresh fruit, such as berries, sliced bananas, or peaches
- 1/4 cup granola
- 1/4 teaspoon cinnamon

Instructions:

1. In a glass or bowl, layer the yogurt, fruit, granola, and cinnamon.
2. Repeat the layers.
3. Enjoy!

Total time: 5 minutes

Servings: 1

Tips:

- Use a low-fat or fat-free yogurt to reduce the calories and saturated fat in your parfait.
- Choose your favorite fresh fruit to add sweetness and flavor to your parfait.
- If you want a sweeter parfait, you can add a small amount of sugar or honey.
- You can also add other toppings to your parfait, such as nuts, seeds, or chocolate chips.

Whole-wheat toast with avocado

Ingredients:

- 1 slice whole-wheat bread

- 1/2 avocado, mashed
- 1/4 teaspoon salt
- 1/4 teaspoon black pepper
- Lime juice, to taste (optional)

Instructions:

1. Toast the bread.
2. Spread the mashed avocado on the toast.
3. Sprinkle with salt, pepper, and lime juice, if desired.
4. Enjoy!

Total time: 5 minutes

Servings: 1

Tips:

- Use ripe avocados for the best flavor and texture.

- If you don't have lime juice, you can use lemon juice or another type of citrus juice.
- You can also add other toppings to your toast, such as eggs, cheese, or sprouts.

Peanut butter toast

Ingredients:

- 2 slices whole-wheat bread
- 2 tablespoons natural peanut butter
- 1/4 teaspoon cinnamon (optional)
- 1/4 teaspoon sugar substitute (optional)

Instructions:

1. Spread peanut butter on one slice of bread.
2. Top with cinnamon and sugar substitute, if desired.
3. Place the other slice of bread on top.
4. Cut the toast in half and enjoy!

Total time: 5 minutes

Servings: 1

Tips:

- Use natural peanut butter, which has less sugar and saturated fat than regular peanut butter.
- If you don't have cinnamon, you can use another spice, such as nutmeg or ginger.
- If you don't like banana, you can top your toast with other fruits, such as berries or honey.

- If you don't have sugar substitute, you can use a small amount of honey or maple syrup.

Bagel with cream cheese

Ingredients:

- 1 whole-wheat bagel
- 1 tablespoon light cream cheese
- 1/2 teaspoon cinnamon
- 1/4 teaspoon sugar substitute

Instructions:

1. Split the bagel in half and toast it lightly.
2. Spread the cream cheese on the bagel halves.
3. Sprinkle with cinnamon and sugar substitute.

4. Enjoy!

Total time: 5 minutes

Servings: 1

Tips:

- Use a light cream cheese to reduce the calories and saturated fat.
- If you don't have cinnamon, you can use another spice, such as nutmeg or ginger.
- If you don't have sugar substitute, you can use a small amount of honey or maple syrup.

Whole-wheat cereal with milk

Ingredients:

- 1 cup whole-wheat cereal
- 1 cup milk of choice
- 1/2 cup fresh fruit, such as berries, sliced bananas, or peaches

Instructions:

1. Combine the cereal and milk in a bowl.
2. Stir until the cereal is softened.
3. Top with the fresh fruit and enjoy!

Total time: 5 minutes

Servings: 1

Tips:

- Use a low-fat or fat-free milk to reduce the calories and saturated fat in your cereal.
- Choose your favorite fresh fruit to add sweetness and flavor to your cereal.
- If you want a sweeter cereal, you can add a small amount of sugar or honey.

Lunch Recipes

Grilled chicken salad with avocado and nuts

Ingredients:

- 1/2 cup cooked chicken breast, grilled or baked
- 1/2 cup chopped romaine lettuce

- 1/4 cup chopped cucumber
- 1/4 cup chopped tomato
- 1/4 cup chopped avocado
- 1 tablespoon chopped nuts (such as almonds, walnuts, or pecans)
- 1 tablespoon olive oil
- 1 tablespoon balsamic vinegar
- 1/2 teaspoon salt
- 1/4 teaspoon black pepper

Instructions:

1. In a large bowl, combine the chicken, lettuce, cucumber, tomato, avocado, and nuts.
2. In a small bowl, whisk together the olive oil, balsamic vinegar, salt, and pepper.
3. Pour the dressing over the salad and toss to coat.
4. Serve immediately.

Total time: 15 minutes

Servings: 2

Tips:

- For a lower-fat option, use fat-free or low-fat dressing.
- To add more flavor, you can add other ingredients to the salad, such as cooked bacon, sausage, or ham.
- You can also make this salad ahead of time and store it in the refrigerator for up to 24 hours.

Lentil soup

Ingredients:

- 1 tablespoon olive oil
- 1/2 cup chopped onion
- 2 cloves garlic, minced
- 1 teaspoon ground cumin
- 1/2 teaspoon turmeric

- 1/2 teaspoon salt
- 1/4 teaspoon black pepper
- 6 cups chicken or vegetable broth
- 1 cup brown lentils, rinsed and sorted
- 1 (14.5 ounce) can diced tomatoes, undrained
- 1 (15 ounce) can black beans, rinsed and drained
- 1/2 cup chopped fresh cilantro
- Juice of 1 lime

Instructions:

1. Heat the olive oil in a large pot over medium heat. Add the onion and cook until softened, about 5 minutes. Add the garlic, cumin, turmeric, salt, and pepper and cook for 1 minute more.
2. Add the broth, lentils, tomatoes, black beans, and cilantro to the pot. Bring to a boil, then reduce heat to low and simmer for 30 minutes, or until the lentils are soft.
3. Stir in the lime juice and serve hot.

Total time: 45 minutes

Servings: 6

Tips:

- For a thicker soup, mash some of the lentils with a fork before serving.
- You can also add other vegetables to the soup, such as carrots, celery, or potatoes.
- This soup can be made ahead of time and stored in the refrigerator for up to 3 days.

Salmon with roasted vegetables

Ingredients:

- 2 (6-ounce) salmon fillets
- 1 tablespoon olive oil
- 1 teaspoon salt

- 1/2 teaspoon black pepper
- 1 red onion, chopped
- 1 red bell pepper, chopped
- 1 yellow bell pepper, chopped
- 1 zucchini, chopped
- 1 (14.5 ounce) can diced tomatoes, undrained
- 1/4 cup chopped fresh basil

Instructions:

1. Preheat the oven to 400 degrees F (200 degrees C).
2. Brush the salmon filets with olive oil and season with salt and pepper.
3. Place the salmon filets in a baking dish and top with the vegetables.
4. Drizzle the vegetables with the juice from the diced tomatoes.
5. Bake for 20 minutes, or until the salmon is cooked through and the vegetables are tender.
6. Garnish with fresh basil and serve hot.

Total time: 30 minutes

Servings: 4

Tips:

- For a healthier option, use wild salmon instead of farmed salmon.
- You can also add other vegetables to the dish, such as carrots, potatoes, or mushrooms.
- This dish can be made ahead of time and stored in the refrigerator for up to 24 hours.

Hard-boiled eggs with whole-wheat toast

Ingredients:

- 6 large eggs
- 1 slice whole-wheat toast
- 1 tablespoon butter

- Salt and pepper to taste

Instructions:

1. Place the eggs in a single layer in a saucepan.
2. Cover the eggs with cold water.
3. Bring the water to a boil over high heat.
4. Once the water is boiling, cover the pan, remove from heat, and let the eggs sit for 12 minutes.
5. Drain the hot water and run cold water over the eggs until they are cool enough to handle.
6. Peel the eggs and slice them in half.
7. Spread the butter on the toast and season with salt and pepper.
8. Top the toast with the sliced eggs and serve.

Total time: 20 minutes

Servings: 2

Tips:

- For a lower-fat option, use light butter or margarine.
- You can also add other toppings to the toast, such as cheese, avocado, or tomato.
- This dish can be made ahead of time and stored in the refrigerator for up to 24 hours.

Chicken stir-fry

Ingredients:

- 1 tablespoon olive oil
- 1 pound boneless, skinless chicken breasts, cut into 1-inch pieces

- 1/2 teaspoon salt
- 1/4 teaspoon black pepper
- 1/2 cup chopped onion
- 1 red bell pepper, chopped
- 1 green bell pepper, chopped
- 1 cup broccoli florets
- 1/2 cup snow peas
- 1/4 cup low-sodium soy sauce
- 1 tablespoon rice vinegar
- 1 tablespoon cornstarch
- 1/4 cup water

Instructions:

1. Heat the olive oil in a large skillet or wok over medium-high heat.
2. Add the chicken and cook until browned on all sides.
3. Season with salt and pepper.
4. Add the onion, bell peppers, broccoli, and snow peas to the skillet.
5. Cook for 5-7 minutes, or until the vegetables are tender-crisp.
6. In a small bowl, whisk together the soy sauce, rice vinegar, cornstarch, and water.

7. Add the soy sauce mixture to the skillet and cook for 1-2 minutes, or until the sauce thickens.
8. Serve immediately.

Total time: 20 minutes

Servings: 4

Tips:

- For a lower-fat option, use lean chicken breast or turkey breast.
- You can also add other vegetables to the stir-fry, such as carrots, mushrooms, or zucchini.
- This dish can be made ahead of time and stored in the refrigerator for up to 24 hours.

Lentil burgers

Ingredients:

- 1 cup cooked lentils
- 1/2 cup chopped onion
- 1/4 cup chopped carrot
- 1/4 cup chopped celery
- 1 egg
- 1/4 cup bread crumbs
- 1 tablespoon olive oil
- 1 teaspoon salt
- 1/2 teaspoon black pepper

Instructions:

1. Preheat the oven to 375 degrees F (190 degrees C).

2. In a large bowl, combine the lentils, onion, carrot, celery, egg, bread crumbs, olive oil, salt, and pepper.
3. Mix well to combine.
4. Form the mixture into 4 patties.
5. Place the patties on a baking sheet and bake for 15-20 minutes, or until cooked through.
6. Serve hot.

Total time: 30 minutes

Servings: 4

Tips:

- For a healthier option, use whole-wheat bread crumbs.
- You can also add other vegetables to the burgers, such as mushrooms, zucchini, or squash.
- These burgers can be made ahead of time and stored in the refrigerator for up to 24 hours.

Black bean soup

Ingredients:

- 1 tablespoon olive oil
- 1/2 cup chopped onion
- 1 clove garlic, minced
- 1 teaspoon ground cumin
- 1/2 teaspoon chili powder
- 1/4 teaspoon salt
- 1/4 teaspoon black pepper
- 1 (15 ounce) can black beans, rinsed and drained
- 1 (14.5 ounce) can diced tomatoes, undrained
- 1/2 cup vegetable broth
- 1/4 cup chopped fresh cilantro

Instructions:

1. Heat the olive oil in a large pot over medium heat.
2. Add the onion and cook until softened, about 5 minutes.
3. Add the garlic, cumin, chili powder, salt, and pepper and cook for 1 minute more.
4. Add the black beans, diced tomatoes, vegetable broth, and cilantro to the pot.
5. Bring to a boil, then reduce heat to low and simmer for 20 minutes, or until the flavors have melded.
6. Serve hot.

Total time: 35 minutes

Servings: 6

Tips:

- For a thicker soup, mash some of the beans with a fork before serving.
- You can also add other vegetables to the soup, such as carrots, celery, or potatoes.

- This soup can be made ahead of time and stored in the refrigerator for up to 3 days.

Salad sandwich

Ingredients:

- 2 slices whole-wheat bread
- 1/2 cup mixed greens
- 1/4 cup shredded carrots
- 1/4 cup cucumber, chopped
- 1/4 cup tomato, chopped
- 1 tablespoon light mayonnaise
- 1/2 teaspoon Dijon mustard
- Salt and pepper to taste

Instructions:

1. Spread the mayonnaise and mustard on one slice of bread.

2. Top with the mixed greens, carrots, cucumber, tomato, and salt and pepper to taste.
3. Top with the other slice of bread.
4. Cut the sandwich in half and serve.

Total time: 10 minutes

Servings: 1

Tips:

- For a lower-calorie option, use light mayonnaise and mustard.
- You can also add other vegetables to the salad, such as avocado, sprouts, or radishes.
- This sandwich can be made ahead of time and stored in the refrigerator for up to 24 hours.

Pasta salad

Ingredients:

- 1 pound whole-wheat pasta
- 1/2 cup chopped red onion
- 1/2 cup chopped green bell pepper
- 1/2 cup chopped cucumber
- 1/2 cup chopped cherry tomatoes
- 1/4 cup chopped black olives
- 1/4 cup grated Parmesan cheese
- 1/4 cup olive oil
- 2 tablespoons red wine vinegar
- 1 teaspoon dried oregano
- 1/2 teaspoon salt
- 1/4 teaspoon black pepper

Instructions:

1. Cook the pasta according to the package directions.
2. Drain the pasta and rinse it with cold water.

3. In a large bowl, combine the pasta, red onion, green bell pepper, cucumber, cherry tomatoes, black olives, Parmesan cheese, olive oil, red wine vinegar, oregano, salt, and pepper.
4. Toss to coat.
5. Serve chilled.

Total time: 30 minutes

Servings: 6

Tips:

- For a lower-fat option, use light olive oil and Parmesan cheese.
- You can also add other vegetables to the salad, such as carrots, celery, or zucchini.
- This salad can be made ahead of time and stored in the refrigerator for up to 24 hours

Quinoa salad

Ingredients:

- 1 cup quinoa
- 2 cups water
- 1/2 cup chopped red onion
- 1/2 cup chopped cucumber
- 1/2 cup chopped tomato
- 1/4 cup chopped black olives
- 1/4 cup chopped parsley
- 1/4 cup olive oil
- 2 tablespoons red wine vinegar
- 1 teaspoon dried oregano
- 1/2 teaspoon salt
- 1/4 teaspoon black pepper

Instructions:

1. Rinse the quinoa in a fine-mesh strainer until the water runs clear.
2. In a medium saucepan, combine the quinoa and water. Bring to a boil over high heat, then reduce heat to low, cover, and simmer for 15 minutes, or

until the quinoa is cooked through and
the water is absorbed.
3. Remove the quinoa from the heat and
let it cool slightly.
4. In a large bowl, combine the quinoa, red
onion, cucumber, tomato, black olives,
parsley, olive oil, red wine vinegar,
oregano, salt, and pepper.
5. Toss to coat.
6. Serve chilled.

Total time: 30 minutes

Servings: 6

Tips:

- For a lower-fat option, use light olive oil.
- You can also add other vegetables to the
  salad, such as carrots, celery, or
  zucchini.
- This salad can be made ahead of time
  and stored in the refrigerator for up to
  24 hours.

Chicken and vegetable soup

Ingredients:

- 1 tablespoon olive oil
- 1 pound boneless, skinless chicken breasts, cut into 1-inch pieces
- 1/2 teaspoon salt
- 1/4 teaspoon black pepper
- 1/2 cup chopped onion
- 1 carrot, chopped
- 1 celery stalk, chopped
- 1 (14.5 ounce) can diced tomatoes, undrained
- 1 (15 ounce) can low-sodium chicken broth
- 1/2 teaspoon dried thyme
- 1/4 teaspoon dried basil
- 1/4 cup chopped fresh parsley

Instructions:

1. Heat the olive oil in a large pot over medium heat.

2. Add the chicken and cook until browned on all sides.
3. Season with salt and pepper.
4. Add the onion, carrot, and celery to the pot and cook until softened, about 5 minutes.
5. Add the diced tomatoes, chicken broth, thyme, basil, and parsley to the pot.
6. Bring to a boil, then reduce heat to low, cover, and simmer for 20 minutes, or until the chicken is cooked through.
7. Serve hot.

Total time: 35 minutes

Servings: 6

Tips:

- For a lower-fat option, use skinless chicken breasts.
- You can also add other vegetables to the soup, such as zucchini, squash, or mushrooms.
- This soup can be made ahead of time and stored in the refrigerator for up to 3 days.

Beef stew

Ingredients:

- 2 tablespoons olive oil
- 2 pounds beef stew meat, cut into 1-inch cubes
- 1 teaspoon salt
- 1/2 teaspoon black pepper
- 1 onion, chopped
- 2 carrots, chopped
- 2 celery stalks, chopped
- 2 tablespoons tomato paste
- 1 (14.5 ounce) can diced tomatoes, undrained
- 1 (15 ounce) can beef broth
- 1/2 teaspoon dried thyme
- 1/4 teaspoon dried basil
- 1/4 cup chopped fresh parsley

Instructions:

1. Heat the olive oil in a large pot over medium heat.

2. Add the beef and cook until browned on all sides.
3. Season with salt and pepper.
4. Add the onion, carrot, and celery to the pot and cook until softened, about 5 minutes.
5. Add the tomato paste and cook for 1 minute more.
6. Add the diced tomatoes, beef broth, thyme, basil, and parsley to the pot.
7. Bring to a boil, then reduce heat to low, cover, and simmer for 2 hours, or until the beef is tender.
8. Serve hot.

Total time: 2 hours and 30 minutes

Servings: 6

Tips:

- For a lower-fat option, use lean beef stew meat.

- You can also add other vegetables to the stew, such as potatoes, zucchini, or squash.
- This stew can be made ahead of time and stored in the refrigerator for up to 3 days.

Fish tacos

Ingredients:

- 1 pound white fish fillets, such as cod, tilapia, or halibut
- 1 tablespoon olive oil
- 1/2 teaspoon salt
- 1/4 teaspoon black pepper
- 1/2 cup shredded cabbage
- 1/4 cup chopped red onion
- 1/4 cup chopped cilantro
- 1 lime, juiced

- 4 (6-inch) whole-wheat tortillas

Instructions:

1. Preheat the oven to 400 degrees F (200 degrees C).
2. In a bowl, combine the fish, olive oil, salt, and pepper.
3. Spread the fish in a single layer on a baking sheet.
4. Bake for 10-12 minutes, or until the fish is cooked through.
5. While the fish is cooking, combine the cabbage, red onion, cilantro, and lime juice in a bowl.
6. Heat the tortillas in a hot pan or microwave.
7. To assemble the tacos, place a piece of fish in a tortilla.
8. Top with the cabbage mixture and serve immediately.

Total time: 20 minutes

Servings: 4

Tips:

- For a lower-fat option, use skinless fish filets.
- You can also add other vegetables to the cabbage mixture, such as carrots, celery, or zucchini.
- This recipe can be made ahead of time and stored in the refrigerator for up to 24 hours.

Lentil loaf

Ingredients:

- 1 cup brown lentils, rinsed and picked over
- 1 (14.5 ounce) can diced tomatoes, undrained
- 1 (15 ounce) can kidney beans, rinsed and drained
- 1/2 cup chopped onion

- 1/2 cup chopped green bell pepper
- 1/4 cup chopped celery
- 1/4 cup chopped fresh parsley
- 1 egg, beaten
- 1/4 cup bread crumbs
- 1 teaspoon dried thyme
- 1/2 teaspoon salt
- 1/4 teaspoon black pepper

Instructions:

1. Preheat oven to 350 degrees F (175 degrees C).
2. In a large bowl, combine the lentils, diced tomatoes, kidney beans, onion, bell pepper, celery, parsley, egg, bread crumbs, thyme, salt, and pepper.
3. Mix well.
4. Pour the mixture into a greased 9x5 inch loaf pan.
5. Bake for 50-60 minutes, or until a toothpick inserted into the center comes out clean.
6. Let cool for 10 minutes before slicing and serving.

Total time: 1 hour and 10 minutes

Servings: 6

Tips:

- For a lower-fat option, use fat-free or low-fat ingredients.
- You can also add other vegetables to the loaf, such as carrots, zucchini, or squash.
- This loaf can be made ahead of time and stored in the refrigerator for up to 3 days.

Quiche

Ingredients:

- 1 (9-inch) unbaked pie crust
- 1 cup milk
- 1/2 cup shredded cheddar cheese
- 1/4 cup grated Parmesan cheese

- 1/4 cup chopped onion
- 1/4 cup chopped green bell pepper
- 1/4 cup chopped mushrooms
- 1/4 teaspoon salt
- 1/8 teaspoon black pepper
- 2 large eggs

Instructions:

1. Preheat the oven to 350 degrees F (175 degrees C).
2. In a medium bowl, whisk together the milk, cheddar cheese, Parmesan cheese, onion, bell pepper, mushrooms, salt, and pepper.
3. In a separate bowl, whisk together the eggs.
4. Pour the egg mixture into the pie crust.
5. Pour the milk mixture over the egg mixture.
6. Bake for 30-35 minutes, or until the quiche is set and the cheese is melted.
7. Let cool for 10 minutes before serving.

Total time: 1 hour

Servings: 6

Tips:

- For a lower-fat option, use fat-free or low-fat ingredients.
- You can also add other vegetables to the quiche, such as broccoli, zucchini, or squash.
- This quiche can be made ahead of time and stored in the refrigerator for up to 24 hours.

Soup and sandwich

Ingredients:

- **Soup:**
  - 1 tablespoon olive oil
  - 1/2 cup chopped onion

- 1/2 cup chopped carrots
- 1/2 cup chopped celery
- 1 teaspoon dried thyme
- 1/2 teaspoon salt
- 1/4 teaspoon black pepper
- 4 cups chicken broth
- 1 (15 ounce) can diced tomatoes, undrained
- 1 cup cooked chicken, shredded
- 1/2 cup cooked brown rice
- 1/4 cup shredded cheddar cheese

- **Sandwich:**
  - 2 slices whole-wheat bread
  - 1 tablespoon mayonnaise
  - 1/4 cup shredded lettuce
  - 1/4 tomato, sliced
  - 1/4 hard-boiled egg, sliced

Instructions:

1. Soup:
   1. Heat the olive oil in a large pot over medium heat.

2. Add the onion, carrots, and celery and cook until softened, about 5 minutes.
3. Add the thyme, salt, and pepper and cook for 1 minute more.
4. Add the chicken broth, diced tomatoes, cooked chicken, and brown rice and bring to a boil.
5. Reduce heat to low and simmer for 15 minutes, or until the vegetables are tender.
6. Stir in the shredded cheddar cheese and serve.
2. Sandwich:
   1. Spread mayonnaise on one slice of bread.
   2. Top with lettuce, tomato, and hard-boiled egg.
   3. Place the other slice of bread on top.
   4. Cut the sandwich in half and serve.

Total time: 30 minutes

Servings: 4

Tips:

- For a lower-fat option, use fat-free or low-fat ingredients.
- You can also add other vegetables to the soup, such as broccoli, zucchini, or squash.
- This soup can be made ahead of time and stored in the refrigerator for up to 24 hours.
- For a lower-fat option, use light butter or margarine.
- You can also use whole-wheat bread.
- This sandwich can be made ahead of time and stored in the refrigerator for up to 24 hours.

Salad with grilled chicken

Ingredients:

- 1 cup cooked chicken breast, grilled or roasted
- 1/2 cup chopped romaine lettuce
- 1/2 cup chopped cucumber
- 1/4 cup chopped tomato
- 1/4 cup chopped red onion
- 1 tablespoon olive oil
- 2 tablespoons balsamic vinegar
- 1 teaspoon Dijon mustard
- 1/2 teaspoon salt
- 1/4 teaspoon black pepper

Instructions:

1. In a large bowl, combine the chicken, lettuce, cucumber, tomato, red onion, olive oil, balsamic vinegar, Dijon mustard, salt, and pepper.
2. Toss to coat.
3. Serve immediately.

Total time: 15 minutes

Servings: 2

Tips:

- For a lower-fat option, use skinless chicken breast.
- You can also add other vegetables to the salad, such as carrots, celery, or zucchini.
- This salad can be made ahead of time and stored in the refrigerator for up to 24 hours.

Salad with tuna

Ingredients:

- 1 can (12 ounces) tuna, drained
- 1/4 cup light mayonnaise

- 1/4 cup chopped celery
- 1/4 cup chopped onion
- 1 tablespoon lemon juice
- 1/2 teaspoon salt
- 1/4 teaspoon black pepper
- 1/4 cup chopped walnuts (optional)

Instructions:

1. In a medium bowl, combine the tuna, light mayonnaise, celery, onion, lemon juice, salt, and pepper.
2. Mix well.
3. If desired, stir in the walnuts.
4. Serve on lettuce leaves or whole-wheat bread.

Total time: 10 minutes

Servings: 2

Tips:

- For a lower-fat option, use light mayonnaise or fat-free Greek yogurt.

- You can also add other vegetables to the salad, such as carrots, cucumbers, or tomatoes.
- This salad can be made ahead of time and stored in the refrigerator for up to 24 hours.

Pasta with marinara sauce

Ingredients:

- 1 pound whole-wheat pasta
- 1 (28 ounce) can whole peeled tomatoes, crushed by hand
- 1/4 cup chopped onion
- 4 cloves garlic, minced
- 1 teaspoon dried oregano
- 1/2 teaspoon salt
- 1/4 teaspoon black pepper
- 1/4 cup chopped fresh basil

Instructions:

1. Bring a large pot of salted water to a boil.
2. Add the pasta and cook according to the package directions.
3. While the pasta is cooking, heat 1 tablespoon of olive oil in a large skillet over medium heat.
4. Add the onion and cook until softened, about 5 minutes.
5. Add the garlic and cook for 1 minute more.
6. Add the crushed tomatoes, oregano, salt, and pepper.
7. Bring to a simmer and cook for 15 minutes, or until the sauce has thickened.
8. Stir in the basil and remove from heat.
9. Drain the pasta and add it to the sauce.
10. Toss to coat.
11. Serve immediately.

Total time: 30 minutes

Servings: 4

Tips:

- For a lower-fat option, use light olive oil or fat-free Greek yogurt.
- You can also add other vegetables to the sauce, such as carrots, zucchini, or squash.
- This dish can be made ahead of time and stored in the refrigerator for up to 24 hours.

Quinoa with black beans and vegetables

Ingredients:

- 1 cup quinoa
- 2 cups vegetable broth
- 1 (15 ounce) can black beans, rinsed and drained
- 1 red bell pepper, diced
- 1 green bell pepper, diced
- 1 onion, diced

- 2 cloves garlic, minced
- 1 teaspoon ground cumin
- 1/2 teaspoon chili powder
- 1/4 teaspoon salt
- 1/4 teaspoon black pepper
- 1/4 cup chopped fresh cilantro

Instructions:

1. Rinse the quinoa in a fine-mesh sieve until the water runs clear.
2. In a medium saucepan, combine the quinoa, vegetable broth, black beans, red bell pepper, green bell pepper, onion, garlic, cumin, chili powder, salt, and pepper.
3. Bring to a boil over high heat, then reduce heat to low, cover, and simmer for 20 minutes, or until the quinoa is cooked through and the liquid is absorbed.
4. Stir in the cilantro and serve.

Total time: 30 minutes

Servings: 4

Tips:

- For a lower-fat option, use fat-free or low-fat broth.
- You can also add other vegetables to the quinoa, such as carrots, zucchini, or squash.
- This dish can be made ahead of time and stored in the refrigerator for up to 24 hours.

Omelet with vegetables

Ingredients:

- 2 large eggs
- 1 tablespoon water
- 1/4 teaspoon salt
- 1/8 teaspoon black pepper
- 1 tablespoon olive oil
- 1/2 cup chopped onion

- 1/2 cup chopped green bell pepper
- 1/4 cup chopped mushrooms
- 1/4 cup shredded cheddar cheese

Instructions:

1. In a medium bowl, whisk together the eggs, water, salt, and pepper.
2. Heat the olive oil in a large nonstick skillet over medium heat.
3. Add the onion and bell pepper and cook until softened, about 5 minutes.
4. Add the mushrooms and cook for 2 minutes more.
5. Pour the egg mixture into the skillet and cook until set, about 2 minutes per side.
6. Sprinkle the cheese and cook until melted, about 1 minute more.
7. Fold the omelet in half and serve.

Total time: 15 minutes

Servings: 2

Tips:

- For a lower-fat option, use fat-free or low-fat cheese.
- You can also add other vegetables to the omelet, such as carrots, zucchini, or squash.
- This dish can be made ahead of time and stored in the refrigerator for up to 24 hours.

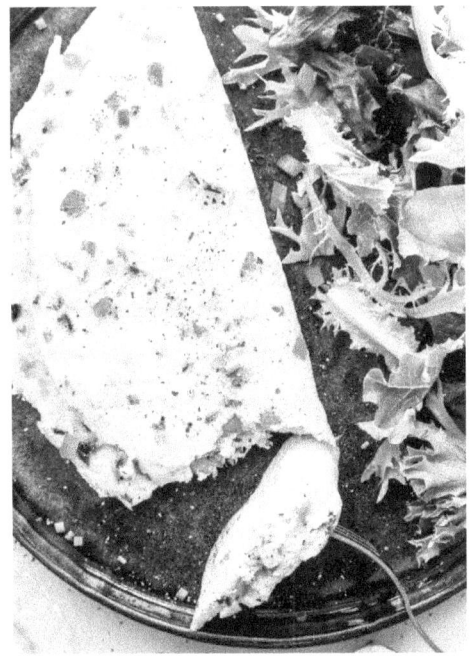

Dinner

Grilled Salmon with Roasted Vegetables

Ingredients:

- 1 (1-pound) salmon fillet, skin on
- 1 tablespoon olive oil
- 1 teaspoon salt
- 1/2 teaspoon black pepper
- 1 red onion, chopped
- 2 carrots, chopped
- 1 zucchini, chopped
- 1 (15 ounce) can black beans, rinsed and drained
- 1/2 cup chopped fresh cilantro

Instructions:

1. Preheat the oven to 400 degrees F (200 degrees C).
2. Brush the salmon filet with olive oil and season with salt and pepper.
3. Place the salmon filet on a baking sheet lined with parchment paper.
4. Roast the salmon in the preheated oven for 15-20 minutes, or until cooked through.
5. While the salmon is roasting, roast the vegetables in a large skillet over medium heat until tender.
6. Once the salmon is cooked, flake it with a fork.
7. Serve the salmon over the roasted vegetables and top with black beans and cilantro.

Total time: 30 minutes

Servings: 2

Tips:

- For a lower-fat option, use fat-free or low-fat broth.
- You can also add other vegetables to the salmon, such as carrots, zucchini, or squash.
- This dish can be made ahead of time and stored in the refrigerator for up to 24 hours.

Turkey Meatballs with Spaghetti Squash

Ingredients:

- 1 pound ground turkey
- 1/2 cup bread crumbs
- 1/4 cup grated Parmesan cheese
- 1 egg
- 1 teaspoon dried oregano

- 1/2 teaspoon garlic powder
- 1/4 teaspoon salt
- 1/8 teaspoon black pepper
- 1 (15 ounce) can crushed tomatoes
- 1 (15 ounce) can tomato sauce
- 1/2 cup water
- 1 spaghetti squash, halved and seeded

Instructions:

1. Preheat the oven to 375 degrees F (190 degrees C).
2. In a large bowl, combine ground turkey, bread crumbs, Parmesan cheese, egg, oregano, garlic powder, salt, and pepper. Mix well.
3. Form the mixture into 1-inch meatballs.
4. In a large skillet, heat 1 tablespoon of olive oil over medium heat. Add the meatballs and cook until browned on all sides.
5. In a large baking dish, combine the crushed tomatoes, tomato sauce, and water. Stir to combine.
6. Add the meatballs to the baking dish and bake for 30 minutes, or until cooked through.

7. While the meatballs are cooking, prepare the spaghetti squash. Cut the squash in half lengthwise and remove the seeds. Place the squash halves cut side down on a baking sheet and bake for 30 minutes, or until tender.
8. When the squash is cooked, use a fork to scrape the flesh into strands.
9. Serve the meatballs over the spaghetti squash.

Total time: 1 hour

Servings: 4

Tips:

- For a lower-fat option, use fat-free or low-fat ground turkey.
- You can also add other vegetables to the meatballs, such as spinach, mushrooms, or zucchini.
- This dish can be made ahead of time and stored in the refrigerator for up to 24 hours.

Shrimp Scampi with Zucchini Noodles

Ingredients:

- 1 pound large shrimp, peeled and deveined
- 1 tablespoon olive oil
- 1/2 cup white wine
- 1/4 cup chicken broth
- 1/4 cup grated Parmesan cheese
- 1/4 teaspoon salt
- 1/8 teaspoon black pepper
- 1/4 cup chopped fresh parsley
- 1 pound zucchini, spiralized

Instructions:

1. Heat the olive oil in a large skillet over medium heat.
2. Add the shrimp and cook until pink and cooked through, about 2 minutes per side.

3. Remove the shrimp from the skillet and set aside.
4. To the same skillet, add the white wine, chicken broth, Parmesan cheese, salt, and pepper. Bring to a simmer and cook for 2 minutes, or until the sauce has thickened slightly.
5. Stir in the parsley and shrimp.
6. Serve immediately over zucchini noodles.

Total time: 15 minutes

Servings: 4

Tips:

- For a lower-fat option, use fat-free or low-fat chicken broth.
- You can also add other vegetables to the sauce, such as mushrooms, spinach, or zucchini.
- This dish can be made ahead of time and stored in the refrigerator for up to 24 hours.

Grilled Chicken Fajitas with Vegetables

Ingredients:

- 1 pound boneless, skinless chicken breasts, cut into 1-inch strips
- 1 tablespoon olive oil
- 1 teaspoon chili powder
- 1/2 teaspoon cumin
- 1/4 teaspoon salt
- 1/8 teaspoon black pepper
- 1 red bell pepper, sliced
- 1 green bell pepper, sliced
- 1 onion, sliced
- 10 (6-inch) flour tortillas
- 1/2 cup shredded cheddar cheese
- 1/4 cup chopped fresh cilantro
- Lime wedges, for serving

Instructions:

1. Preheat the grill to medium heat.

2. In a large bowl, combine chicken, olive oil, chili powder, cumin, salt, and pepper. Toss to coat.
3. Grill chicken for 5-7 minutes per side, or until cooked through.
4. While the chicken is grilling, heat a large skillet over medium heat. Add the bell peppers and onion and cook until softened, about 5 minutes.
5. To assemble the fajitas, place a tortilla on a plate. Top with chicken, vegetables, cheese, and cilantro. Squeeze lime juice over the top. Fold the tortilla in half and enjoy!

Total time: 20 minutes

Servings: 4

Tips:

- For a lower-fat option, use fat-free or low-fat cheese.
- You can also add other vegetables to the fajitas, such as mushrooms, zucchini, or squash.

- This dish can be made ahead of time and stored in the refrigerator for up to 24 hours.

Black Bean Burgers with Sweet Potato Fries

Ingredients:

- 1 (15 ounce) can black beans, rinsed and drained
- 1/2 cup cooked brown rice
- 1/4 cup oats
- 1/4 cup chopped onion
- 1/4 cup chopped red bell pepper
- 1/4 cup chopped cilantro
- 1 egg
- 1 teaspoon chili powder
- 1/2 teaspoon cumin
- 1/4 teaspoon salt

- 1/8 teaspoon black pepper
- 1 tablespoon olive oil
- 1 sweet potato, peeled and cut into fries

Instructions:

1. Preheat the oven to 400 degrees F (200 degrees C).
2. In a large bowl, combine black beans, brown rice, oats, onion, bell pepper, cilantro, egg, chili powder, cumin, salt, and pepper. Mix well.
3. Form the mixture into 4 patties.
4. Heat the olive oil in a large skillet over medium heat. Add the patties and cook for 5-7 minutes per side, or until cooked through.
5. While the patties are cooking, prepare the sweet potato fries. Toss the sweet potato fries with olive oil and salt. Spread the fries on a baking sheet and bake for 20-25 minutes, or until golden brown and crispy.
6. Serve the patties on a bun with the sweet potato fries and your favorite toppings.

Total time: 40 minutes

Servings: 4

Tips:

- For a lower-fat option, use fat-free or low-fat cheese.
- You can also add other vegetables to the burgers, such as spinach, mushrooms, or zucchini.
- This dish can be made ahead of time and stored in the refrigerator for up to 24 hours.

Chicken Parmesan with Whole-Wheat Pasta

Ingredients:

- 6 boneless, skinless chicken breasts
- 1/2 cup whole wheat flour
- 1 teaspoon salt
- 1/2 teaspoon black pepper
- 1 egg, beaten
- 1 cup panko bread crumbs
- 1/2 cup grated Parmesan cheese
- 1/4 cup olive oil
- 1 (28 ounce) can crushed tomatoes
- 1 (15 ounce) can tomato sauce
- 1/2 cup grated mozzarella cheese
- 1/4 cup chopped fresh basil
- 12 ounces whole-wheat spaghetti

Instructions:

1. Preheat the oven to 400 degrees F (200 degrees C).

2. Pound the chicken breasts to 1/4-inch thickness.
3. In a shallow dish, combine the flour, salt, and pepper. In another shallow dish, beat the egg. In a third shallow dish, combine the panko bread crumbs and Parmesan cheese.
4. Dredge the chicken breasts in the flour mixture, then the egg, then the panko bread crumb mixture.
5. Heat the olive oil in a large skillet over medium heat. Add the chicken breasts and cook for 5-7 minutes per side, or until golden brown and cooked through.
6. In a small bowl, combine the crushed tomatoes, tomato sauce, and mozzarella cheese.
7. Spread half of the tomato sauce mixture in the bottom of a 9x13 inch baking dish. Top with the chicken breasts. Spread the remaining tomato sauce mixture over the chicken breasts.
8. Bake for 20 minutes, or until the chicken is cooked through and the cheese is melted and bubbly.

9. While the chicken is baking, cook the whole-wheat spaghetti according to the package directions.
10. Serve the chicken parmesan with the whole-wheat spaghetti and garnish with fresh basil.

Total time: 45 minutes

Servings: 6

Tips:

- For a lower-fat option, use fat-free or low-fat cheese.
- You can also add other vegetables to the sauce, such as mushrooms, spinach, or zucchini.
- This dish can be made ahead of time and stored in the refrigerator for up to 24 hours.

Salmon with Roasted Asparagus

Ingredients:

- 2 (6 ounce) salmon fillets, skin on
- 1 tablespoon olive oil
- 1/2 teaspoon salt
- 1/4 teaspoon black pepper
- 1 pound asparagus, trimmed
- 1/4 cup grated Parmesan cheese
- 1/4 cup chopped fresh parsley

Instructions:

1. Preheat the oven to 400 degrees F (200 degrees C).
2. In a small bowl, combine the olive oil, salt, and pepper. Rub the mixture all over the salmon filets.
3. Place the salmon filets on a baking sheet lined with parchment paper.
4. Roast the salmon for 12-15 minutes, or until cooked through.
5. While the salmon is roasting, prepare the asparagus.

6. Toss the asparagus with olive oil and salt.
7. Spread the asparagus on a baking sheet and roast for 10-12 minutes, or until tender.
8. To serve, top the salmon with the roasted asparagus, Parmesan cheese, and parsley.

Total time: 30 minutes

Servings: 2

Tips:

- For a lower-fat option, use fat-free or low-fat cheese.
- You can also add other vegetables to the asparagus, such as mushrooms, spinach, or zucchini.
- This dish can be made ahead of time and stored in the refrigerator for up to 24 hours.

Tofu Stir-Fry with Brown Rice

Ingredients:

- 1 block extra-firm tofu, pressed and crumbled
- 1 tablespoon soy sauce
- 1 tablespoon rice vinegar
- 1 teaspoon sesame oil
- 1/2 teaspoon garlic powder
- 1/4 teaspoon black pepper
- 1/4 cup chopped green onions
- 1/2 cup chopped carrots
- 1/2 cup chopped broccoli
- 1/2 cup cooked brown rice

Instructions:

1. In a medium bowl, combine the tofu, soy sauce, rice vinegar, sesame oil, garlic powder, and black pepper. Mix well to coat.
2. Heat a large skillet or wok over medium heat. Add the tofu mixture and cook, stirring occasionally, for 5-7 minutes, or

until the tofu is cooked through and the vegetables are tender.
3. Stir in the green onions and serve over brown rice.

Total time: 20 minutes

Servings: 4

Tips:

- For a lower-fat option, use fat-free or low-fat soy sauce and rice vinegar.
- You can also add other vegetables to the stir-fry, such as mushrooms, spinach, or zucchini.
- This dish can be made ahead of time and stored in the refrigerator for up to 24 hours.

Chicken Soup with Quinoa

Ingredients:

- 1 tablespoon olive oil
- 1/2 cup chopped onion
- 1/2 cup chopped celery
- 2 carrots, chopped
- 1 (14.5 ounce) can diced tomatoes, undrained
- 1 (10 ounce) can diced tomatoes with green chilies, undrained
- 4 cups chicken broth
- 1 cup quinoa
- 1/2 teaspoon salt
- 1/4 teaspoon black pepper
- 1 (10 ounce) package cooked chicken, shredded
- 1/4 cup chopped fresh parsley

Instructions:

1. Heat the olive oil in a large pot over medium heat. Add the onion, celery, and carrots and cook, stirring occasionally, until softened, about 5 minutes.
2. Add the diced tomatoes, diced tomatoes with green chilies, chicken broth, quinoa, salt, and pepper and bring to a boil.
3. Reduce heat to low, cover, and simmer for 20 minutes, or until the quinoa is cooked through.
4. Stir in the chicken and parsley.
5. Serve hot.

Total time: 30 minutes

Servings: 6

Tips:

- For a lower-fat option, use fat-free or low-fat chicken broth and cheese.
- You can also add other vegetables to the soup, such as mushrooms, spinach, or zucchini.

- This dish can be made ahead of time and stored in the refrigerator for up to 24 hours.

This recipe for Chicken Soup with Quinoa is a healthy and delicious option for pregnant women with gestational diabetes. It is low in sugar and carbohydrates, and it is made with whole grain quinoa. This recipe is also a good source of fiber and protein, which can help to keep blood sugar levels stable.

Lentil Salad with Grilled Chicken

Ingredients:

- 1 cup lentils
- 1 cup water

- 1/2 cup chopped onion
- 1/2 cup chopped celery
- 1/2 cup chopped carrots
- 1/4 cup chopped red bell pepper
- 1/4 cup chopped green bell pepper
- 1/4 cup chopped cucumber
- 1/4 cup chopped tomatoes
- 1/4 cup chopped fresh parsley
- 1/4 cup olive oil
- 2 tablespoons red wine vinegar
- 1 tablespoon Dijon mustard
- 1 teaspoon salt
- 1/2 teaspoon black pepper
- 1/4 teaspoon garlic powder
- 1/4 teaspoon onion powder
- 1/4 teaspoon paprika
- 1/4 teaspoon cayenne pepper
- 1/2 cup grilled chicken, shredded

Instructions:

1. Cook the lentils according to the package directions.
2. While the lentils are cooking, heat the olive oil in a large skillet over medium heat. Add the onion, celery, carrots, red bell pepper, and green bell pepper and

cook, stirring occasionally, until softened, about 5 minutes.
3. Add the cucumber, tomatoes, parsley, red wine vinegar, Dijon mustard, salt, pepper, garlic powder, onion powder, paprika, and cayenne pepper to the skillet and stir to combine.
4. Drain the lentils and add them to the skillet. Stir to combine.
5. Serve the salad warm or cold, topped with the grilled chicken.

Total time: 30 minutes

Servings: 6

Black Bean Salad with Quinoa

Ingredients:

- 1 cup quinoa
- 1 cup water
- 1 (15 ounce) can black beans, rinsed and drained
- 1/2 cup chopped red onion
- 1/2 cup chopped green bell pepper
- 1/4 cup chopped cucumber
- 1/4 cup chopped tomatoes
- 1/4 cup chopped fresh parsley
- 1/4 cup olive oil
- 2 tablespoons red wine vinegar
- 1 tablespoon Dijon mustard
- 1 teaspoon salt
- 1/2 teaspoon black pepper
- 1/4 teaspoon garlic powder
- 1/4 teaspoon onion powder
- 1/4 teaspoon paprika
- 1/4 teaspoon cayenne pepper

Instructions:

1. Cook the quinoa according to the package directions.

2. While the quinoa is cooking, heat the olive oil in a large skillet over medium heat. Add the red onion, green bell pepper, and cucumber and cook, stirring occasionally, until softened, about 5 minutes.
3. Add the tomatoes, parsley, red wine vinegar, Dijon mustard, salt, pepper, garlic powder, onion powder, paprika, and cayenne pepper to the skillet and stir to combine.
4. Drain the quinoa and add it to the skillet. Stir to combine.
5. Serve the salad warm or cold, topped with the black beans.

Total time: 30 minutes

Servings: 6

Shrimp Scampi with Whole-Wheat Pasta

Ingredients:

- 1 pound whole-wheat pasta
- 1 pound shrimp, peeled and deveined
- 1/4 cup olive oil
- 1/4 cup butter
- 2 cloves garlic, minced
- 1/2 teaspoon dried oregano
- 1/4 teaspoon red pepper flakes
- 1/4 cup dry white wine
- 1/4 cup chicken broth
- 1/4 cup chopped fresh parsley
- Salt and pepper to taste

Instructions:

1. Cook the pasta according to the package directions.
2. While the pasta is cooking, heat the olive oil and butter in a large skillet over medium heat.
3. Add the shrimp and cook, stirring occasionally, until pink and cooked through, about 2-3 minutes.

4. Add the garlic, oregano, and red pepper flakes and cook for 1 minute more.
5. Add the white wine and chicken broth and bring to a boil.
6. Reduce heat to low and simmer for 5 minutes, or until the sauce has thickened slightly.
7. Stir in the parsley, salt, and pepper.
8. Serve the shrimp scampi over the cooked pasta.

Total time: 30 minutes

Servings: 4

Grilled Chicken Fajitas with Brown Rice

Ingredients:

- 1 pound boneless, skinless chicken breasts, cut into 1-inch strips
- 1 tablespoon olive oil
- 1/2 teaspoon salt
- 1/4 teaspoon black pepper
- 1 onion, chopped
- 1 green bell pepper, chopped
- 1 red bell pepper, chopped
- 1 (10 ounce) can diced tomatoes and green chilies, undrained
- 1/2 cup chopped fresh cilantro
- 12 (6-inch) flour tortillas
- 1 cup cooked brown rice
- Lime wedges, for serving

Instructions:

1. Preheat grill to medium heat.
2. In a large bowl, combine chicken, olive oil, salt, and pepper. Toss to coat.
3. Grill chicken for 5-7 minutes per side, or until cooked through.
4. While chicken is grilling, heat a large skillet over medium heat. Add onion, bell peppers, and diced tomatoes and

green chilies. Cook, stirring occasionally, until vegetables are softened, about 5 minutes.
5. Remove from heat and stir in cilantro.
6. To assemble fajitas, place a tortilla on a flat surface. Top with grilled chicken, vegetables, brown rice, and lime wedges. Roll up and serve.

Total time: 30 minutes

Servings: 6

Black Bean Burgers with Whole-Wheat Buns

Ingredients:

- 1 (15 ounce) can black beans, rinsed and drained
- 1/2 cup whole wheat bread crumbs
- 1/4 cup chopped onion
- 1/4 cup chopped red bell pepper
- 1 egg, beaten
- 1 tablespoon olive oil
- 1 teaspoon chili powder
- 1/2 teaspoon ground cumin
- 1/4 teaspoon salt
- 1/4 teaspoon black pepper
- 4 whole-wheat buns, toasted
- Your favorite toppings, such as lettuce, tomato, avocado, and cheese

Instructions:

1. Preheat the oven to 375 degrees F (190 degrees C).
2. In a large bowl, combine black beans, bread crumbs, onion, bell pepper, egg, olive oil, chili powder, cumin, salt, and pepper. Mix until well combined.
3. Form the mixture into 4 patties.

4. Place the patties on a baking sheet and bake for 15-20 minutes, or until cooked through.
5. Serve on toasted whole-wheat buns with your favorite toppings.

Total time: 30 minutes

Servings: 4

Chicken Parmesan with Spaghetti Squash

Ingredients:

- 1 medium spaghetti squash
- 1 pound boneless, skinless chicken breasts, pounded thin
- 1/2 cup all-purpose flour
- 1/2 cup grated Parmesan cheese
- 1 egg, beaten
- 1/4 teaspoon salt

- 1/4 teaspoon black pepper
- 1/4 cup olive oil
- 1 (15 ounce) can tomato sauce
- 1/2 cup shredded mozzarella cheese

Instructions:

1. Preheat the oven to 400 degrees F (200 degrees C).
2. Cut the spaghetti squash in half lengthwise and remove the seeds. Place the halves cut-side down on a baking sheet and bake for 30-40 minutes, or until tender.
3. While the squash is baking, prepare the chicken. In a shallow dish, combine the flour, Parmesan cheese, egg, salt, and pepper. Dip the chicken in the mixture and coat evenly.
4. Heat the olive oil in a large skillet over medium heat. Add the chicken and cook for 3-4 minutes per side, or until golden brown and cooked through.
5. Spread a layer of tomato sauce in the bottom of a 9x13 inch baking dish. Top with the chicken and then with the mozzarella cheese.

6. Bake for 15-20 minutes, or until the cheese is melted and bubbly.
7. Serve with the cooked spaghetti squash.

Total time: 1 hour and 15 minutes

Servings: 4

Salmon with Roasted Brussels Sprouts

Ingredients:

- 1 pound salmon fillets, skin on
- 1 tablespoon olive oil
- 1 teaspoon salt
- 1/2 teaspoon black pepper
- 1 pound Brussels sprouts, trimmed and halved
- 1/4 cup olive oil

- 1/4 cup balsamic vinegar
- 1 teaspoon dried thyme
- 1/2 teaspoon garlic powder
- 1/4 teaspoon salt
- 1/4 teaspoon black pepper

Instructions:

1. Preheat the oven to 400 degrees F (200 degrees C).
2. In a large bowl, toss the salmon with 1 tablespoon olive oil, salt, and pepper.
3. Place the salmon on a baking sheet and bake for 12-15 minutes, or until cooked through.
4. Meanwhile, in a large bowl, toss the Brussels sprouts with 1/4 cup olive oil, balsamic vinegar, thyme, garlic powder, salt, and pepper.
5. Spread the Brussels sprouts on a baking sheet and roast for 20-25 minutes, or until tender and browned.
6. Serve the salmon with the roasted Brussels sprouts.

Total time: 40 minutes

Servings: 4

Tofu Stir-Fry with Cauliflower Rice

Ingredients:

- 1 head cauliflower, broken into florets
- 1 tablespoon olive oil
- 1/2 onion, chopped
- 2 cloves garlic, minced
- 1 pound extra-firm tofu, pressed and crumbled
- 1/2 cup broccoli florets
- 1/2 cup carrots, chopped
- 1/4 cup snow peas
- 1/4 cup soy sauce
- 1 tablespoon rice vinegar
- 1 teaspoon sesame oil
- 1/2 teaspoon ginger, grated
- 1/4 teaspoon red pepper flakes

- Salt and pepper to taste

Instructions:

1. Prepare the cauliflower rice by pulsing the cauliflower florets in a food processor until they resemble rice.
2. Heat the olive oil in a large skillet or wok over medium heat.
3. Add the onion and garlic and cook, stirring occasionally, until softened, about 5 minutes.
4. Add the tofu and cook, stirring occasionally, until browned, about 5 minutes.
5. Add the broccoli, carrots, snow peas, soy sauce, rice vinegar, sesame oil, ginger, red pepper flakes, salt, and pepper.
6. Cook, stirring occasionally, until the vegetables are tender, about 5 minutes.
7. Serve immediately over the cauliflower rice.

Total time: 25 minutes

Servings: 4

Chicken Soup with Lentils

Ingredients:

- 1 tablespoon olive oil
- 1 onion, chopped
- 2 carrots, chopped
- 2 celery stalks, chopped
- 1 teaspoon dried thyme
- 1/2 teaspoon dried oregano
- 1/4 teaspoon salt
- 1/4 teaspoon black pepper
- 6 cups chicken broth
- 1 cup lentils
- 1/2 cup cooked chicken, shredded
- 1/4 cup chopped fresh parsley

Instructions:

1. Heat the olive oil in a large pot over medium heat.
2. Add the onion, carrots, celery, thyme, oregano, salt, and pepper. Cook, stirring occasionally, until the vegetables are softened, about 5 minutes.
3. Add the chicken broth and lentils. Bring to a boil, then reduce heat to low and simmer for 30 minutes, or until the lentils are soft.
4. Stir in the chicken and parsley. Serve hot.

Total time: 45 minutes

Servings: 6

Black Bean Salad with Cornbread

Ingredients:

- 1 (15 ounce) can black beans, rinsed and drained
- 1 (15 ounce) can corn, drained
- 1/2 cup chopped red onion
- 1/2 cup chopped green bell pepper
- 1/4 cup chopped cilantro
- 1/4 cup olive oil
- 2 tablespoons lime juice
- 1 teaspoon chili powder
- 1/2 teaspoon cumin
- 1/4 teaspoon salt
- 1/4 teaspoon black pepper
- 12 cornbread muffins, crumbled

Instructions:

1. In a large bowl, combine the black beans, corn, red onion, green bell pepper, cilantro, olive oil, lime juice, chili powder, cumin, salt, and pepper.
2. Mix well to combine.
3. Crumble the cornbread muffins over the salad and mix well to combine.
4. Serve immediately.

Total time: 20 minutes

Servings: 6

Vegetarian Recipes

Tofu veggie burgers

Ingredients:

- 1 block extra-firm tofu, pressed and crumbled
- 1/2 cup chopped onion
- 1/2 cup chopped green bell pepper
- 1/4 cup chopped carrots
- 1/4 cup chopped celery
- 1/4 cup cooked quinoa
- 1/4 cup bread crumbs
- 1 egg, beaten
- 1 tablespoon soy sauce
- 1 teaspoon garlic powder
- 1/2 teaspoon onion powder
- 1/4 teaspoon salt
- 1/4 teaspoon black pepper

Instructions:

1. Preheat the oven to 375 degrees F (190 degrees C).
2. In a large bowl, combine the tofu, onion, bell pepper, carrots, celery, quinoa, bread crumbs, egg, soy sauce, garlic powder, onion powder, salt, and pepper. Mix well to combine.
3. Form the mixture into 4 patties.
4. Place the patties on a baking sheet lined with parchment paper.
5. Bake for 20-25 minutes, or until golden brown and cooked through.
6. Serve on whole-wheat buns with your favorite toppings.

Total time: 45 minutes

Servings: 4

Smoothie made with yogurt, fruit, and protein powder

Ingredients:

- 1 cup plain Greek yogurt
- 1 cup unsweetened almond milk
- 1/2 cup frozen berries (any type)
- 1 tablespoon protein powder (optional)

Instructions:

1. Combine all ingredients in a blender and blend until smooth.
2. Pour into a glass and enjoy!

Total time: 5 minutes

Servings: 1

This smoothie is a great way to get a quick and healthy breakfast or snack. It is low in sugar and carbohydrates, and it is a good source of protein, calcium, and fiber. The berries are a good source of antioxidants, and the protein powder can help to keep you feeling full.

Here are some tips for making a gestational diabetes-friendly smoothie:

- Use unsweetened almond milk or another low-carb milk alternative.
- Choose berries that are low in sugar, such as strawberries, raspberries, or blueberries.
- If you are using protein powder, choose a brand that is low in sugar and carbohydrates.
- Avoid adding any added sugar or syrup to your smoothie.
- You can also add other healthy ingredients to your smoothie, such as spinach, kale, or avocado.

Salad with grilled vegetables and chickpeas

Ingredients:

- 1 tablespoon olive oil
- 1 onion, chopped
- 2 carrots, chopped
- 1 zucchini, chopped
- 1 red bell pepper, chopped
- 1 can chickpeas, drained and rinsed
- 1/2 cup chopped fresh parsley
- 1/4 cup balsamic vinegar
- 2 tablespoons olive oil
- 1 teaspoon Dijon mustard
- 1/2 teaspoon salt
- 1/4 teaspoon black pepper

Instructions:

1. Preheat the grill to medium heat.

2. In a large bowl, combine the onion, carrots, zucchini, bell pepper, and chickpeas.
3. Drizzle with olive oil and toss to coat.
4. Grill the vegetables for 10-15 minutes, or until tender.
5. In a small bowl, whisk together the balsamic vinegar, olive oil, Dijon mustard, salt, and pepper.
6. Pour the dressing over the grilled vegetables and toss to coat.
7. Serve immediately, garnished with fresh parsley.

Total time: 30 minutes

Servings: 4

Soup with whole-grain bread

Ingredients:

- 1 tablespoon olive oil
- 1 onion, chopped
- 2 carrots, chopped
- 2 celery stalks, chopped
- 1 teaspoon garlic powder
- 1/2 teaspoon dried thyme
- 1/4 teaspoon salt
- 1/4 teaspoon black pepper
- 4 cups chicken or vegetable broth
- 1 (15 ounce) can diced tomatoes, undrained
- 1 (15 ounce) can black beans, rinsed and drained
- 1 (15 ounce) can corn, drained
- 1/2 cup chopped fresh cilantro
- 1/4 cup chopped fresh parsley
- 4 slices whole-wheat bread, toasted

Instructions:

1. Heat the olive oil in a large pot over medium heat. Add the onion, carrots, celery, garlic powder, thyme, salt, and pepper. Cook, stirring occasionally, until the vegetables are softened, about 5 minutes.
2. Add the broth, tomatoes, black beans, corn, cilantro, and parsley to the pot. Bring to a boil, then reduce heat and simmer for 15 minutes, or until the flavors have blended.
3. Serve hot, with a slice of whole-wheat bread on the side.

Total time: 30 minutes

Servings: 6

Veggie burger on a whole-wheat bun

Ingredients:

- 1 (15 ounce) can black beans, rinsed and drained
- 1 (15 ounce) can corn, drained
- 1/2 cup cooked quinoa
- 1/2 cup chopped onion
- 1/4 cup chopped red bell pepper
- 1/4 cup chopped green bell pepper
- 1/4 cup chopped carrots
- 1/4 cup chopped celery
- 1 egg, beaten
- 1/4 cup bread crumbs
- 1 tablespoon chili powder
- 1 teaspoon cumin
- 1/2 teaspoon salt
- 1/4 teaspoon black pepper
- 4 whole-wheat buns
- Your favorite toppings, such as lettuce, tomato, onion, avocado, and ketchup

Instructions:

1. Preheat the oven to 375 degrees F (190 degrees C).
2. In a large bowl, combine the black beans, corn, quinoa, onion, bell peppers, carrots, celery, egg, bread crumbs, chili powder, cumin, salt, and pepper. Mix well to combine.
3. Form the mixture into 4 patties.
4. Place the patties on a baking sheet lined with parchment paper.
5. Bake for 20-25 minutes, or until golden brown and cooked through.
6. Serve on whole-wheat buns with your favorite toppings.

Total time: 45 minutes

Servings: 4

Lentil soup with brown rice

Ingredients:

- 1 tablespoon olive oil
- 1 onion, chopped
- 2 carrots, chopped
- 2 celery stalks, chopped
- 1 teaspoon garlic powder
- 1/2 teaspoon dried thyme
- 1/4 teaspoon salt
- 1/4 teaspoon black pepper
- 4 cups chicken or vegetable broth
- 1 (15 ounce) can diced tomatoes, undrained
- 1 cup lentils, rinsed and sorted
- 1/2 cup brown rice
- 1/2 cup chopped fresh cilantro
- 1/4 cup chopped fresh parsley

Instructions:

1. Heat the olive oil in a large pot over medium heat. Add the onion, carrots,

celery, garlic powder, thyme, salt, and pepper. Cook, stirring occasionally, until the vegetables are softened, about 5 minutes.

2. Add the broth, tomatoes, lentils, brown rice, cilantro, and parsley to the pot. Bring to a boil, then reduce heat and simmer for 30 minutes, or until the lentils and rice are cooked through.
3. Serve hot.

Total time: 45 minutes

Servings: 6

This soup is a great source of protein, fiber, and complex carbohydrates. It is also low in sugar and fat, making it a healthy option for people with gestational diabetes. The lentils and brown rice are both good sources of complex carbohydrates, which will help to keep you feeling full and satisfied. The vegetables in the soup are a good source of vitamins, minerals, and antioxidants. The cilantro and parsley add a fresh flavor to the soup.

Here are some tips for making a gestational diabetes-friendly lentil soup:

- Use low-sodium broth.
- Rinse the lentils before cooking to remove any excess starch.
- Use brown rice instead of white rice.
- Add a variety of vegetables to the soup, such as carrots, celery, onions, and tomatoes.
- Season the soup with herbs and spices, such as garlic powder, thyme, and salt and pepper.
- Serve the soup with a side of whole-wheat bread or crackers.

Hummus and vegetables

Ingredients:

- 1 (15 ounce) can chickpeas, drained and rinsed
- 1/4 cup tahini
- 1/4 cup lemon juice
- 1/4 cup olive oil
- 2 cloves garlic, minced
- 1 teaspoon salt
- 1/2 teaspoon ground cumin
- 1/4 teaspoon black pepper
- Vegetables of your choice, such as carrots, celery, cucumbers, and bell peppers

Instructions:

1. In a food processor, combine the chickpeas, tahini, lemon juice, olive oil, garlic, salt, and cumin. Process until smooth.
2. Taste and adjust the seasonings as needed.
3. Serve with vegetables of your choice.

Total time: 10 minutes

Servings: 4

Hummus is a great source of protein and fiber, and it is low in sugar and fat. It is a healthy option for people with gestational diabetes. The vegetables in this recipe add a variety of nutrients and flavors.

Here are some tips for making a gestational diabetes-friendly hummus:

- Use whole-wheat pita bread or crackers for dipping.
- Avoid adding any added sugar or syrup to the hummus.
- You can also add other healthy ingredients to the hummus, such as spinach, kale, or avocado.

Tofu stir-fry with vegetables

Ingredients:

- 1 block extra-firm tofu, pressed and crumbled
- 1 tablespoon cornstarch
- 1 tablespoon soy sauce
- 1 tablespoon rice vinegar
- 1 tablespoon sesame oil
- 1 teaspoon minced ginger
- 1 teaspoon minced garlic
- 1/2 cup chopped onion
- 1/2 cup chopped carrots
- 1/2 cup chopped broccoli
- 1/4 cup chopped snow peas
- 1/4 cup chopped red bell pepper
- 1/4 cup chopped green onions
- Salt and pepper to taste

Instructions:

1. In a medium bowl, combine the tofu, cornstarch, soy sauce, rice vinegar, sesame oil, ginger, and garlic. Mix well to coat.
2. Heat a large skillet or wok over medium-high heat. Add the tofu mixture and cook, stirring constantly, until the tofu is golden brown and cooked through.

3. Add the onion, carrots, broccoli, snow peas, and red bell pepper to the skillet. Cook, stirring occasionally, until the vegetables are tender-crisp.
4. Season with salt and pepper to taste.
5. Serve immediately, garnished with green onions.

Total time: 20 minutes

Servings: 4

This stir-fry is a great source of protein and fiber, and it is low in sugar and fat. It is a healthy option for people with gestational diabetes. The vegetables in this recipe add a variety of nutrients and flavors.

Here are some tips for making a gestational diabetes-friendly tofu stir-fry:

- Use extra-firm tofu, which is lower in fat and calories than other types of tofu.
- Press the tofu before cooking to remove excess water.
- Use low-sodium soy sauce and rice vinegar.

- Choose vegetables that are low in carbohydrates, such as broccoli, carrots, and snow peas.
- Serve with brown rice or quinoa for a complete meal.

Lentil pasta with marinara sauce

Ingredients:

- 12 ounces lentil pasta
- 1 jar (28 ounces) marinara sauce
- 1/2 cup grated Parmesan cheese
- 1/4 cup chopped fresh basil
- Salt and pepper to taste

Instructions:

1. Cook the lentil pasta according to the package directions.
2. While the pasta is cooking, heat the marinara sauce in a large saucepan over medium heat.
3. Once the pasta is cooked, drain it and add it to the saucepan with the marinara sauce.
4. Stir to combine and heat through.
5. Serve immediately, topped with Parmesan cheese, basil, salt, and pepper to taste.

Total time: 20 minutes

Servings: 4

Here are some tips for making a gestational diabetes-friendly lentil pasta with marinara sauce:

- Use whole-wheat lentil pasta, which is a good source of fiber.
- Choose a marinara sauce that is low in sugar and fat.
- Serve with a side of vegetables for a complete meal.

Vegetable lasagna

Ingredients:

- 12 lasagna noodles
- 1 tablespoon olive oil
- 1 onion, chopped
- 2 cloves garlic, minced
- 1 (14.5 ounce) can diced tomatoes, undrained
- 1 (15 ounce) can tomato sauce
- 1 teaspoon dried oregano
- 1/2 teaspoon dried basil
- 1/4 teaspoon salt
- 1/4 teaspoon black pepper
- 1 (10 ounce) package frozen spinach, thawed and squeezed dry
- 1 (15 ounce) can black beans, rinsed and drained
- 1/2 cup grated Parmesan cheese

Instructions:

1. Preheat the oven to 375 degrees F (190 degrees C).

2. In a large skillet, heat the olive oil over medium heat. Add the onion and garlic and cook, stirring occasionally, until softened, about 5 minutes.
3. Stir in the diced tomatoes, tomato sauce, oregano, basil, salt, and pepper. Bring to a simmer and cook for 15 minutes, or until the sauce has thickened.
4. In a medium bowl, combine the spinach, black beans, and Parmesan cheese.
5. Spread a thin layer of the tomato sauce in the bottom of a 9x13 inch baking dish. Top with 3 lasagna noodles, overlapping as needed. Spread with half of the spinach mixture and half of the remaining tomato sauce. Repeat layers.
6. Cover with foil and bake for 30 minutes. Uncover and bake for an additional 15 minutes, or until the lasagna is heated through and bubbly.
7. Let stand for 10 minutes before serving.

Total time: 1 hour

Servings: 8

Vegetarian tacos

Ingredients:

- 1 tablespoon olive oil
- 1 onion, chopped
- 1 red bell pepper, chopped
- 1 green bell pepper, chopped
- 1 (15 ounce) can black beans, rinsed and drained
- 1 (15 ounce) can corn, drained
- 1 (10 ounce) can diced tomatoes and green chilies, undrained
- 1 teaspoon chili powder
- 1/2 teaspoon cumin
- 1/4 teaspoon salt
- 1/4 teaspoon black pepper
- 12 corn tortillas
- Your favorite toppings, such as shredded lettuce, chopped tomatoes, shredded cheese, sour cream, and guacamole

Instructions:

1. Heat the olive oil in a large skillet over medium heat. Add the onion, red bell pepper, and green bell pepper and cook, stirring occasionally, until softened, about 5 minutes.
2. Stir in the black beans, corn, diced tomatoes and green chilies, chili powder, cumin, salt, and pepper. Bring to a simmer and cook for 10 minutes, or until the flavors have blended.
3. Warm the tortillas in a microwave or on a griddle.
4. To assemble the tacos, spread some of the black bean mixture on a tortilla and top with your favorite toppings.
5. Serve immediately.

Total time: 25 minutes

Servings: 6

Lentil Salad with Grilled Veggie Patties

Ingredients:

- 1 cup lentils, cooked
- 1/2 cup chopped red onion
- 1/2 cup chopped cucumber
- 1/4 cup chopped tomato
- 1/4 cup chopped green bell pepper
- 1/4 cup chopped fresh parsley
- 2 tablespoons olive oil
- 2 tablespoons balsamic vinegar
- 1 teaspoon Dijon mustard
- 1/2 teaspoon salt
- 1/4 teaspoon black pepper
- 4 veggie patties

Instructions:

1. In a large bowl, combine the lentils, red onion, cucumber, tomato, green bell pepper, and parsley.
2. In a small bowl, whisk together the olive oil, balsamic vinegar, Dijon mustard, salt, and pepper.

3. Pour the dressing over the lentil mixture and toss to coat.
4. Grill the veggie patties according to the package directions.
5. Serve the lentil salad topped with the veggie patties.

Total time: 30 minutes

Servings: 4

Vegetarian Chili with Cornbread

Ingredients:

- 1 tablespoon olive oil
- 1/2 cup chopped onion
- 1/2 cup chopped green bell pepper
- 1 clove garlic, minced
- 1 teaspoon chili powder

- 1/2 teaspoon ground cumin
- 1/4 teaspoon salt
- 1/4 teaspoon black pepper
- 1 (15 ounce) can black beans, rinsed and drained
- 1 (15 ounce) can kidney beans, rinsed and drained
- 1 (14.5 ounce) can diced tomatoes, undrained
- 1 (10 ounce) can diced tomatoes with green chilies, undrained
- 1 cup water
- 1 cup whole wheat elbow macaroni
- 1/2 cup shredded reduced-fat cheddar cheese
- 1/4 cup chopped fresh cilantro
- 1 (8 ounce) package cornbread mix
- 1/2 cup milk
- 1/4 cup vegetable oil

Instructions:

1. Heat the olive oil in a large pot over medium heat. Add the onion, bell pepper, and garlic and cook, stirring occasionally, until softened, about 5 minutes.

2. Add the chili powder, cumin, salt, and pepper and cook for 1 minute more.
3. Stir in the black beans, kidney beans, diced tomatoes, diced tomatoes with green chilies, and water. Bring to a boil, then reduce heat to low and simmer for 15 minutes, or until the flavors have blended.
4. Meanwhile, cook the macaroni according to the package directions, using whole wheat pasta.
5. Drain the macaroni and add it to the chili mixture. Stir until combined.
6. Stir in the cheese and cilantro.
7. Preheat the oven to 400 degrees F (200 degrees C).
8. In a medium bowl, combine the cornbread mix, milk, and oil. Mix until just combined.
9. Pour the batter into a greased 8x8 inch baking dish.
10. Bake for 20-25 minutes, or until a toothpick inserted into the center comes out clean.
11. Serve the chili with the cornbread.

Total time: 1 hour

Servings: 6

Tips:

- For a lower-fat option, use fat-free or low-fat chili beans and cheese.
- You can also add other vegetables to the chili, such as mushrooms, spinach, or zucchini.
- This dish can be made ahead of time and stored in the refrigerator for up to 24 hours.

This recipe for Vegetarian Chili with Cornbread is a healthy and delicious option for pregnant women with gestational diabetes. It is low in sugar and carbohydrates, and it is made with whole wheat pasta and reduced-fat cheese. This recipe is also a good source of fiber and protein, which can help to keep blood sugar levels stable.

Vegetarian Chili Mac

Ingredients:

- 1 tablespoon olive oil
- 1/2 cup chopped onion
- 1/2 cup chopped green bell pepper
- 1 clove garlic, minced
- 1 teaspoon chili powder
- 1/2 teaspoon ground cumin
- 1/4 teaspoon salt
- 1/4 teaspoon black pepper
- 1 (15 ounce) can black beans, rinsed and drained
- 1 (15 ounce) can kidney beans, rinsed and drained
- 1 (14.5 ounce) can diced tomatoes, undrained
- 1 (10 ounce) can diced tomatoes with green chilies, undrained
- 1 cup water
- 1 cup elbow macaroni
- 1/2 cup shredded cheddar cheese
- 1/4 cup chopped fresh cilantro

Instructions:

1. Heat the olive oil in a large pot over medium heat. Add the onion, bell pepper, and garlic and cook, stirring occasionally, until softened, about 5 minutes.
2. Add the chili powder, cumin, salt, and pepper and cook for 1 minute more.
3. Stir in the black beans, kidney beans, diced tomatoes, diced tomatoes with green chilies, and water. Bring to a boil, then reduce heat to low and simmer for 15 minutes, or until the flavors have blended.
4. Meanwhile, cook the macaroni according to the package directions.
5. Drain the macaroni and add it to the chili mixture. Stir until combined.
6. Stir in the cheese and cilantro.
7. Serve hot.

Total time: 30 minutes

Servings: 6

Tips:

This recipe for Vegetarian Chili Mac is a healthy and delicious option for pregnant women with gestational diabetes. It is low in sugar and carbohydrates, and it is made with whole wheat pasta and reduced-fat cheese. This recipe is also a good source of fiber and protein, which can help to keep blood sugar levels stable.

Desterts

Chocolate Avocado Brownies

Ingredients:

- 1 ripe avocado, mashed
- 1/2 cup unsweetened cocoa powder
- 1/2 cup sugar substitute
- 2 eggs
- 1 teaspoon vanilla extract
- 1/4 cup all-purpose flour
- 1/4 teaspoon baking powder
- 1/4 teaspoon salt

Instructions:

1. Preheat the oven to 350 degrees F (175 degrees C). Grease and flour an 8-inch square baking pan.

2. In a large bowl, combine the avocado, cocoa powder, sugar substitute, eggs, and vanilla extract. Beat until smooth.
3. In a separate bowl, whisk together the flour, baking powder, and salt. Gradually add to the wet ingredients, mixing until just combined.
4. Pour the batter into the prepared pan and bake for 25-30 minutes, or until a toothpick inserted into the center comes out clean.
5. Let cool completely before cutting into squares and serving.

Total time: 1 hour

Servings: 9

Tips:

- Use a sugar substitute that is approved for use during pregnancy.
- If you are concerned about the fat content of the avocado, you can use a light or reduced-fat version.

- You can also add in some chocolate chips or other toppings to the brownies for a bit of extra flavor.
- Enjoy!

Peanut Butter Banana Ice Cream

Ingredients:

- 2 frozen bananas, sliced
- 1/2 cup peanut butter
- 1/4 cup milk of choice
- 1/4 cup sugar substitute
- 1 teaspoon vanilla extract

Instructions:

1. In a food processor, combine the frozen bananas, peanut butter, milk, sugar substitute, and vanilla extract. Process until smooth.
2. Pour the ice cream into a serving bowl and enjoy!

Total time: 10 minutes

Servings: 2

Tips:

- Use a sugar substitute that is approved for use during pregnancy.
- If you are concerned about the fat content of the milk, you can use a non-fat or low-fat version.
- You can also add in some chocolate chips or other toppings to the ice cream for a bit of extra flavor.
- Enjoy!

Apple Crisp

Ingredients:

- 6 cups peeled, cored, and sliced apples
- 1/2 cup sugar substitute
- 1/4 cup all-purpose flour
- 1/4 teaspoon ground cinnamon
- 1/4 teaspoon ground nutmeg
- 1/4 teaspoon salt
- 1/4 cup butter, melted
- 1/4 cup chopped walnuts (optional)

Instructions:

1. Preheat the oven to 375 degrees F (190 degrees C). Grease a 9x13 inch baking dish.
2. In a large bowl, combine the apples, sugar substitute, flour, cinnamon, nutmeg, and salt. Toss to coat.
3. Pour the apple mixture into the prepared baking dish. Drizzle with melted butter and sprinkle with walnuts, if desired.

4. Bake for 30-35 minutes, or until the apples are tender and the topping is golden brown.
5. Serve warm with a scoop of ice cream or whipped cream.

Total time: 1 hour

Servings: 6

Tips:

- Use a sugar substitute that is approved for use during pregnancy.
- If you are concerned about the fat content of the butter, you can use a light or reduced-fat version.
- You can also add in some other fruits, such as pears or berries, to the crisp for a bit of extra flavor.
- Enjoy!

Pumpkin Pie

Ingredients:

- 1 (15-ounce) can pumpkin puree
- 1/2 cup sugar substitute
- 1/4 cup all-purpose flour
- 1/4 teaspoon ground cinnamon
- 1/4 teaspoon ground ginger
- 1/4 teaspoon ground nutmeg
- 1/4 teaspoon salt
- 1 egg
- 1/2 cup milk of choice
- 1 teaspoon vanilla extract

Instructions:

1. Preheat the oven to 350 degrees F (175 degrees C).
2. Grease and flour a 9-inch pie plate.
3. In a large bowl, combine the pumpkin puree, sugar substitute, flour, cinnamon, ginger, nutmeg, and salt. Beat until smooth.

4. In a separate bowl, whisk together the egg, milk, and vanilla extract. Add to the pumpkin mixture and beat until just combined.
5. Pour the filling into the prepared pie plate and bake for 45-50 minutes, or until a toothpick inserted into the center comes out clean.
6. Let cool completely before serving.

Total time: 1 hour

Servings: 6

Tips:

- Use a sugar substitute that is approved for use during pregnancy.
- If you are concerned about the fat content of the milk, you can use a non-fat or low-fat version.
- You can also add in some whipped cream or ice cream to the pie for a bit of extra sweetness.
- Enjoy!

Cheesecake

Ingredients:

- 1 (9-inch) graham cracker crust
- 1 (8-ounce) package cream cheese, softened
- 1/2 cup sugar substitute
- 2 eggs
- 1 teaspoon vanilla extract

Instructions:

Preheat the oven to 350 degrees F (175 degrees C).

In a large bowl, beat together the cream cheese and sugar substitute until smooth. Beat in the eggs one at a time, then stir in the vanilla extract.

Pour the batter into the prepared crust and bake for 30-35 minutes, or until the center is set.

Let cool completely before serving.

Total time: 1 hour

Servings: 8

Coconut macaroons

Ingredients:

- 1 cup unsweetened shredded coconut
- 1/2 cup sugar substitute
- 1/4 teaspoon salt
- 4 large egg whites
- 1 teaspoon vanilla extract

Instructions:

1. Preheat the oven to 300 degrees F (150 degrees C).

2. Line a baking sheet with parchment paper.
3. In a medium bowl, combine the coconut, sugar substitute, and salt.
4. In a separate bowl, beat the egg whites until stiff peaks form.
5. Gently fold the egg whites into the coconut mixture until just combined.
6. Drop by rounded tablespoons onto the prepared baking sheet.
7. Bake for 25-30 minutes, or until golden brown.
8. Let cool completely on the baking sheet before serving.

Total time: 45 minutes

Servings: 12

Baked pears

Ingredients:

- 4 ripe pears
- 1/4 cup sugar substitute
- 1/4 teaspoon ground cinnamon
- 1/4 teaspoon ground nutmeg
- 1/4 teaspoon ground ginger
- 1/4 teaspoon salt
- 1 tablespoon butter, melted
- 1 tablespoon lemon juice

Instructions:

1. Preheat the oven to 375 degrees F (190 degrees C).
2. Core the pears and cut them in half lengthwise.
3. In a small bowl, combine the sugar substitute, cinnamon, nutmeg, ginger, and salt.
4. Rub the spice mixture all over the cut sides of the pears.

5. Place the pears in a baking dish cut side up. Drizzle with melted butter and lemon juice.
6. Bake for 30-35 minutes, or until the pears are tender when pierced with a fork.
7. Serve warm or at room temperature.

Total time: 1 hour

Servings: 4

Peanut butter fudge

Ingredients:

- 1 cup sugar substitute
- 1/2 cup unsweetened cocoa powder
- 1/4 cup creamy peanut butter
- 1/4 cup milk of choice

- 1/4 teaspoon vanilla extract

Instructions:

1. In a medium saucepan, combine the sugar substitute and cocoa powder. Stir over medium heat until melted and smooth.
2. Remove from heat and stir in the peanut butter, milk, and vanilla extract.
3. Pour the mixture into a greased 8x8 inch baking dish.
4. Refrigerate for at least 2 hours, or until set.
5. Cut into squares and enjoy!

Total time: 30 minutes

Servings: 9

Blueberry Crumble

Ingredients:

- 6 cups fresh or frozen blueberries
- 1/4 cup sugar substitute
- 1/4 teaspoon ground cinnamon
- 1/4 teaspoon ground nutmeg
- 1/4 teaspoon salt
- 1/4 cup all-purpose flour
- 1/4 cup rolled oats
- 1/4 cup brown sugar
- 1/4 cup butter, melted

Instructions:

1. Preheat the oven to 375 degrees F (190 degrees C).
2. In a large bowl, combine the blueberries, sugar substitute, cinnamon, nutmeg, and salt. Toss to coat.
3. Pour the blueberry mixture into a greased 9x13 inch baking dish.

4. In a small bowl, combine the flour, oats, brown sugar, and melted butter. Mix until crumbly.
5. Sprinkle the crumble topping over the blueberry mixture.
6. Bake for 30-35 minutes, or until the topping is golden brown and the blueberries are bubbly.
7. Let cool slightly before serving.

Total time: 1 hour

Servings: 6

Chocolate protein balls

Ingredients:

- 1 cup rolled oats
- 1/2 cup peanut butter

- 1/4 cup unsweetened cocoa powder
- 1/4 cup sugar substitute
- 1/4 cup honey
- 1/4 cup milk of choice
- 1/4 teaspoon vanilla extract
- 1/4 cup chocolate chips (optional)

Instructions:

1. In a large bowl, combine the oats, peanut butter, cocoa powder, sugar substitute, honey, milk, and vanilla extract. Mix until well combined.
2. Stir in the chocolate chips, if desired.
3. Roll the mixture into small balls and place them on a baking sheet lined with parchment paper.
4. Refrigerate for at least 2 hours, or until set.
5. Enjoy!

Total time: 30 minutes

Servings: 12

Lemon poppy seed muffins

Ingredients:

- 1 cup almond flour
- 1/2 cup coconut flour
- 1/2 cup sugar substitute
- 1/2 teaspoon baking soda
- 1/2 teaspoon baking powder
- 1/4 teaspoon salt
- 1 tablespoon poppy seeds
- 1/4 cup melted butter
- 1 egg
- 1/2 cup unsweetened almond milk
- 1/4 cup lemon juice
- 1 teaspoon lemon extract

Instructions:

1. Preheat the oven to 350 degrees F (175 degrees C). Line a 12-cup muffin tin with paper liners.
2. In a large bowl, whisk together the almond flour, coconut flour, sugar

substitute, baking soda, baking powder, and salt.
3. In a separate bowl, whisk together the melted butter, egg, almond milk, lemon juice, and lemon extract.
4. Add the wet ingredients to the dry ingredients and stir until just combined. Do not overmix.
5. Fold in the poppy seeds.
6. Pour the batter into the prepared muffin tins and bake for 20-25 minutes, or until a toothpick inserted into the center comes out clean.
7. Let cool in the pan for a few minutes before removing to a wire rack to cool completely.

Total time: 45 minutes

Servings: 12

Cinnamon roasted almonds

Ingredients:

- 1 cup whole almonds
- 1 tablespoon ground cinnamon
- 1/4 teaspoon salt
- 1 tablespoon olive oil

Instructions:

1. Preheat the oven to 350 degrees F (175 degrees C).
2. In a medium bowl, combine the almonds, cinnamon, and salt. Toss to coat.
3. Drizzle with olive oil and toss to coat again.
4. Spread the almonds in a single layer on a baking sheet.
5. Bake for 15-20 minutes, or until the almonds are golden brown and fragrant.
6. Let cool completely before serving.

Total time: 35 minutes

Servings: 4

Banana oat cookies

Ingredients:

- 2 ripe bananas, mashed
- 1/2 cup sugar substitute
- 1/4 cup unsweetened applesauce
- 1/4 cup peanut butter
- 1 egg
- 1 teaspoon vanilla extract
- 1 cup rolled oats
- 1/2 cup all-purpose flour
- 1/2 teaspoon baking soda
- 1/4 teaspoon salt
- 1/4 cup chocolate chips (optional)

Instructions:

1. Preheat the oven to 350 degrees F (175 degrees C).
2. In a large bowl, combine the mashed bananas, sugar substitute, applesauce, peanut butter, egg, and vanilla extract. Mix until well combined.
3. In a separate bowl, whisk together the oats, flour, baking soda, and salt.
4. Add the dry ingredients to the wet ingredients and stir until just combined. Do not overmix.
5. Stir in the chocolate chips, if desired.
6. Drop by rounded tablespoons onto ungreased baking sheets.
7. Bake for 10-12 minutes, or until golden brown.
8. Let cool on baking sheets for a few minutes before transferring to a wire rack to cool completely.

Total time: 30 minutes

Servings: 12

Berry Sorbet

Ingredients:

- 2 cups fresh or frozen berries (such as strawberries, raspberries, blueberries, blackberries)
- 1/2 cup sugar substitute
- 1/4 cup water
- 1 tablespoon lemon juice

Instructions:

1. In a blender, combine the berries, sugar substitute, water, and lemon juice. Blend until smooth.
2. Pour the mixture into an ice cream maker and freeze according to the manufacturer's instructions.
3. Once the sorbet is frozen, scoop it into bowls and enjoy!

Total time: 30 minutes

Servings: 4

Chocolate avocado mousse

Ingredients:

- 1 large avocado, peeled, pitted, and mashed
- 1/4 cup unsweetened cocoa powder
- 1/4 cup sugar substitute
- 1/4 cup milk of choice
- 1/4 teaspoon vanilla extract

Instructions:

1. In a blender, combine the avocado, cocoa powder, sugar substitute, milk, and vanilla extract. Blend until smooth.

2. Pour the mousse into serving bowls and refrigerate for at least 2 hours, or until set.
3. Enjoy!

Total time: 15 minutes

Servings: 4

Resources and More Information for Gestational Diabetes

Environmental Working Group, a nonprofit environmental watchdog group, examines data on pesticide residues provided by the U.S. Department of Agriculture and the Food and Drug Administration.

It generates a ranking of the top and worst pesticide doses discovered in industrial crops each year.

These lists might help you choose which foods are considered safe enough to be purchased conventionally and which should be purchased organically to reduce your exposure to pesticides. Although they are safe to purchase, these fruits and vegetables should still be carefully washed.

The list is updated annually, and you can find it online at EWG.org/FoodNews

Where can I get more information about gestational diabetes?

- The American Diabetes Association
- The National Institute of Child Health and Human Development
- The March of Dimes

GOODLUCK!